Curbside Consultation
in Uveitis

49 Clinical Questions

Curbside Consultation in Ophthalmology
SERIES

SERIES EDITOR, DAVID F. CHANG, MD

Curbside Consultation
in Uveitis

49 Clinical Questions

EDITOR

C. Stephen Foster, MD, FACS, FACR

Clinical Professor of Ophthalmology, Harvard Medical School
President & CEO, Massachusetts Eye Research & Surgery Institution
Founder & President, Ocular Immunology & Uveitis Foundation
Cambridge, Massachusetts

ASSOCIATE EDITORS

E. Mitchel Opremcak, MD

Clinical Associate Professor, The Ohio State University College of Medicine
Department of Ophthalmology
The Retina Group
Columbus, Ohio

David M. Hinkle, MD

Massachusetts Eye Research and Surgery Institution
Cambridge, Massachusetts

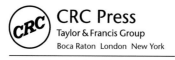

CRC Press
Taylor & Francis Group
Boca Raton London New York

CRC Press is an imprint of the
Taylor & Francis Group, an **informa** business

First published 2012 by SLACK Incorporated

Published 2024 by CRC Press
2385 NW Executive Center Drive, Suite 320, Boca Raton FL 33431

and by CRC Press
4 Park Square, Milton Park, Abingdon, Oxon, OX14 4RN

CRC Press is an imprint of Taylor & Francis Group, LLC

Library of Congress Cataloging-in-Publication Data

Curbside consultation in uveitis : 49 clinical questions / editor, C. Stephen Foster ; associate editors, E. Mitchel Opremcak, David M. Hinkle.
    p. ; cm. -- (Curbside consultation in ophthalmology series)
  Uveitis
  Includes bibliographical references and index.
  ISBN 978-1-55642-998-9 (alk. paper)
  I. Foster, C. Stephen (Charles Stephen), 1942- II. Opremcak, E. Mitchel. III. Hinkle, David M. IV. Title: Uveitis.
V. Series: Curbside consultation in ophthalmology series.
  [DNLM: 1. Uveitis--diagnosis. 2. Uveitis--therapy. WW 240]
  LC classification not assigned
  617.7'3--dc23
                              2011048248

ISBN: 9781556429989 (pbk)
ISBN: 9781003523710 (ebk)

DOI: 10.1201/9781003523710

Dedication

To all of those who have gone before us; we all stand on the shoulders of others. We are indebted to the visionaries who have dedicated themselves to the study of uveitis and to the care of those with uveitis.

Contents

Acknowledgments

We, the editor and associate editors, would like to thank the numerous contributors without whom this book would not have been possible. Additionally, we would like to acknowledge Dr. Sana S. Siddique for her unstinting dedication to editorial assistance and organizational efforts in bringing this collaborated project to completion.

About the Editor

C. Stephen Foster, MD, FACS, FACR was born and raised in West Virginia, received his Bachelor of Science Degree in Chemistry at Duke University, with Distinction and Phi Beta Kappa in 1965, and received his Doctor of Medicine Degree at Duke University Medical Center, in 1969, being elected to Alpha Omega Alpha. He trained in Internal Medicine at Duke University Hospital from 1969 to 1970, and at the National Heart and Lung Institute, at the National Institutes of Health in Bethesda, Maryland, from 1970 to 1972, during which time he also taught Internal Medicine, with an appointment as Instructor in Medicine at the George Washington University Hospital in Washington, DC. In 1972, Dr. Foster entered his Ophthalmology Residency training program at Washington University (Barnes Hospital), in St. Louis, Missouri, and having completed that in 1975, traveled to Boston to do 2 additional Fellowship trainings in Cornea and External Diseases, and in Ocular Immunology. He completed this training in 1977 and was invited to join the full-time faculty of the Department of Ophthalmology of Harvard Medical School, where he was a member of the Cornea Service and Director of the Residency Training Program at the Massachusetts Eye and Ear Infirmary. He began his independent research in 1977 and has since been continuously funded by grants from the National Institutes of Health.

After 30 years on the full time faculty of Massachusetts Eye and Ear Infirmary, he decided to establish his own private practice—The Massachusetts Eye Research and Surgery Institution, a state of the art 12,000 square foot practice with its own chemotherapy infusion suite and phlebotomy lab. Dr. Foster continues to direct a research laboratory at the Massachusetts Eye Research and Surgery Institution (MERSI), through the support of his newly created research foundation, The Ocular Immunology and Uveitis Foundation, and continues his teaching activities and training fellows as a Clinical Professor of Ophthalmology at Harvard Medical School. He has also authored over 600 published papers and 5 textbooks.

About the Associate Editors

E. Mitchel Opremcak, MD did his residency and chief residency in ophthalmology at Ohio State University and his fellowships in both Uveitis and Retina at the Massachusetts Eye and Ear Infirmary at Harvard Medical School. In 1988, he joined the faculty at Ohio State University where he was the Director of the Ocular Immunology and Uveitis Service, and is currently a Clinical Associate Professor. Dr. Opremcak founded both The Retina Group and The Eye Center of Columbus, Ohio. In addition, he has served as President of The Ohio Ophthalmology Society, Chairman of the American Academy of Ophthalmology, and has authored many manuscripts, chapters, and books on the topic including *Uveitis: A Clinical Manual for Ocular Inflammation.*

David M. Hinkle, MD acted as a resident and chief resident in ophthalmology at Tulane University. Dr. Hinkle also completed a fellowship in Ocular Immunology and Uveitis at Harvard Medical School, Massachusetts Eye and Ear Infirmary, and Massachusetts Eye Research and Surgery Institution (MERSI), and has been a staff physician at MERSI since 2007. He has written many papers on a variety of topics within the field of uveitis and contributed chapters to several publications devoted to ocular inflammatory disease.

Contributing Authors

Esen K. Akpek, MD (Question 20)
Associate Professor of Ophthalmology
Rheumatology Director
Ocular Surface Disease and Dry Eye Clinic
Associate Director
Johns Hopkins Jerome L. Greene Sjögren's
  Syndrome Center Director
The Wilmer Eye Institute
Johns Hopkins University
Baltimore, Maryland

Amro Ali, MD (Question 9)
Uveitis Fellow
Oregon Health & Science University
Casey Eye Institute
Portland, Oregon

Sofia Androudi, MD (Question 18)
Lecturer
University of Thessalia
Larissa, Greece

Stephen D. Anesi, MD (Question 19)
Staff Physician, Massachusetts Eye
  Research & Surgery Institution
Cambridge, Massachusetts

William Ayliffe, FRCS, PhD (Question 34)
Consultant Ophthalmologist
National Health Service and Lister Hospital
London, England

Neal P. Barney, MD (Question 1)
Associate Professor
Department of Ophthalmology and
  Visual Sciences
University of Wisconsin
School of Medicine and Public Health
University of Wisconsin Hospital
  and Clinics
Madison, Wisconsin

Periklis Brazitikos, MD (Question 18)
Associate Professor of Ophthalmology
University of Thessaloniki
Thessaloniki, Greece

Nicholas J. Butler, MD (Question 24)
Assistant Professor of Ophthalmology
Johns Hopkins University School of
  Medicine
The Wilmer Eye Institute
Baltimore, Maryland

Margarita Calonge, MD (Question 35)
Professor of Ophthalmology
Instituto Universitario de Oftalmobiologia
  Aplicada
Universidad de Valladolid
Valladolid, Spain

Chi-Chao Chan, MD (Question 21)
Chief, Immunopathology Section
Laboratory of Immunology
Chief, NEI Histology Core
National Eye Institute
Bethesda, Maryland

David S. Chu, MD (Question 23)
Clinical Associate Professor of
  Ophthalmology
New Jersey Medical School—UMDNJ
Newark, New Jersey
Metropolitan Eye Research &
  Surgery Institute
Palisades Park, New Jersey

*Emmett T. Cunningham Jr, MD, PhD, MPH
  (Question 27)*
Director, The Uveitis Service
California Pacific Medical Center,
Adjunct Clinical Professor of
  Ophthalmology
Stanford University School of Medicine
West Coast Retina Medical Group
San Francisco, California

Mark S. Dacey, MD (Question 15)
Colorado Retina Associates, PC
Assistant Professor of Ophthalmology
University of Colorado School of Medicine
Denver, Colorado

Janet L. Davis, MD (Question 36)
Professor of Ophthalmology
Bascom Palmer Eye Institute
University of Miami School of Medicine
Miami, Florida

Khayyam Durrani, MD (Chapter 44)
Chief Clinical Fellow
Massachusetts Eye Research &
   Surgery Institution
Harvard Medical School
Cambridge, Massachusetts

Jose Cuevas Francisco III, MD (Question 49)
Comprehensive Ophthalmologist
Medical Retina and Uveitis
Rizal Eye Center
RAKKK Prophet Medical Center, Inc.
Gumaca, Quezon Province, Philippines

Debra A. Goldstein, MD, FRCSC
   (Question 25)
Director Uveitis Service
Professor of Ophthalmology
Department of Ophthalmology and Visual
   Sciences
University of Illinois at Chicago
Chicago, Illinois

Arusha Gupta, MD (Question 20)
Clinical Fellow
Cornea and External Disease Division
The Wilmer Eye Institute
Johns Hopkins University
Baltimore, Maryland

Gary N. Holland, MD (Question 26)
Jack H. Skirball Professor of Ocular
   Inflammatory Diseases
Chief, Cornea and Uveitis Division
Department of Ophthalmology
David Geffen School of Medicine at UCLA
Jules Stein Eye Institute
Los Angeles, California

John J. Huang, MD (Question 45)
Associate Professor
Residency Program Director
Director of Ocular Immunology and
   Uveitis
Co-Director of Vitreo-Retina
Director of Clinical Trials and
   Translational Research
Director of Ocular Trauma
Yale University
New Haven, Connecticut

Muhammad Kashif Israr, MBBS (Question 22)
Research Fellow
Massachusetts Eye Research & Surgery
   Institution
Cambridge, Massachusetts

Henry J. Kaplan, MD (Question 14)
Evans Professor of Ophthalmology &
   Visual Sciences
University of Louisville School of
   Medicine
Department of Ophthalmology &
   Visual Sciences
Kentucky Lions Eye Center
Louisville, Kentucky

John H. Kempen, MD, PhD (Question 42)
Associate Professor of Ophthalmology and
   Epidemiology
Director, Ocular Inflammation Service,
   Scheie Eye Institute
Director, Ophthalmic Epidemiology and
   International Ophthalmology
Senior Scholar, Center for Clinical
   Epidemiology and Biostatistics
University of Pennsylvania School of
   Medicine
Philadelphia, Pennsylvania

Olivia L. Lee, MD (Question 11)
Assistant Professor of Ophthalmology
Keck School of Medicine
University of Southern California
Doheny Eye Institute
Los Angeles, California

Phuc Lehoang, MD, PhD (Question 38)
Professor and Chair of Ophthalmology
Universite Pierre et Marie Curie
Department of Ophthalmology
Pitie-Salpetriere Hospital
Paris, France

Erik Letko, MD (Question 30)
Corneal Consultants of Colorado
Denver, Colorado

Zhi Jian Li, MD (Question 45)
Professor
Department of Ophthalmology
First Affiliate Hospital
Harbin Medical University
Vice Director of Cataract and Cornea
  Diseases
Nangang, Harbin, China

*Sue Lightman, PhD, FRCP, FRCOphth
  (Question 7)*
Professor of Clinical Ophthalmology
UCL/Institute of Ophthalmology and
  Moorfields Eye Hospital
London, United Kingdom

Dorine Makhoul, MD (Question 16)
Resident in Ophthalmology
Univeristy Hospital CHU Saint Pierre
Depatement of Ophthalmology
Brussels, Belgium

*Annal Dhananjayan Meleth, MD, MS
  (Question 21)*
Clinical Fellow
Medical Retina, Uveitis and Ocular
  Immunology
National Eye Institute
Bethesda, Maryland

Elisabetta Miserocchi, MD (Question 39)
Ocular Immunology and Uveitis Service
Department of Ophthalmology
Scientific Institute San Raffaele
Milan, Italy

Lama Mulki, MD (Question 28)
Clinical Research Fellow in Uveitis
Ocular Immunology and Uveitis
  Foundation
Massachusetts Eye Research & Surgery
  Institution
Cambridge, Massachusetts

Ron Neumann, MD (Question 4)
Chairperson
International Symposium of Ocular
  Pharmacology and Therapeutics,
  Specializing in Ocular Inflammatory
  Diseases
Ramat HaSharon, Israel

Quan Dong Nguyen, MD, MSc (Question 3)
Associate Professor of Ophthalmology
Diseases of the Retina and Vitreous,
  and Uveitis
Wilmer Eye Institute
Johns Hopkins University School of
  Medicine and Hospital
Baltimore, Maryland

*Suzanne Katrina V. Palafox, MD
  (Question 31)*
Visiting Consultant Staff
Department of Ophthalmology
Asian Hospital and Medical Center
Manila, Philippines

John Randolph, MD (Question 14)
House Officer
University of Louisville School of Medicine
Department of Ophthalmology &
  Visual Sciences
Kentucky Lions Eye Center
Louisville, Kentucky

Narsing A. Rao, MD (Question 17)
Professor of Ophthalmology and
  Pathology
University of Southern California
Department of Ophthalmology
Doheny Eye Institute
Los Angeles, California

Russell W. Read, MD, PhD (Question 6)
Associate Professor of Ophthalmology
    and Pathology
Director, Uveitis and Ocular Inflammatory
    Diseases Service
Director, Ophthalmology Residency
    Program
Director, UAB Ocular Immunology
    Laboratory
University of Alabama at Birmingham
Birmingham, Alabama

Alejandro Rodríguez-García, MD (Question 8)
Director of the Ocular Immunology &
    Uveitis Service
Instituto de Oftalmologia y Ciencias
    Visuales
Escuela de Medicina
TEC Salud, del Sistema Tecnologico
    de Monterrey
Monterrey, Nuevo León, Mexico

Manolette R. Roque, MD, MBA (Question 41)
Section Chief, Uveitis
Department of Ophthalmology
St. Luke's Medical Center Global City
Asian Hospital and Medical Center
Manila, Philippines

James T. Rosenbaum, MD (Question 9)
Professor of Ophthalmology, Medicine,
    and Cell Biology
Edward E. Rosenbaum Professor of
    Inflammation Research
Chief, Division of Arthritis & Rheumatic
    Diseases
Director, Uveitis Clinic
Oregon Health & Science University
Casey Eye Institute
Portland, Oregon

Aniki Rothova, MD, PhD (Question 10)
Professor of Ophthalmology
Erasmus Medical Center
Rotterdam, Netherlands

Maite Sainz de la Maza, MD (Question 47)
Associate Professor of Ophthalmology
Clinical Institute of Ophthalmology
Barcelona Central University
Barcelona, Spain

C. Michael Samson, MD, MBA (Question 11)
Associate Professor, New York Medical
    College
The New York Eye & Ear Infirmary
Ophthalmology Subspecialist in Ocular
    Inflammation & Uveitis
Co-Director, Uveitis Service, The New
    York Eye & Ear Infirmary
Director, Uveitis Fellowship, The New
    York Eye & Ear Infirmary
New York, New York

H. Nida Sen, MD, MHSc (Questions 21 and 46)
Director, Uveitis and Ocular Immunology
    Fellowship Program
National Eye Institute
Bethesda, MD
Associate Clinical Professor
Department of Ophthalmology
The George Washington University
Washington, DC

Yasir J. Sepah, MBBS (Question 3)
Postdoctoral Research Fellow
Retinal Imaging Research and
    Reading Center
Wilmer Eye Institute
Johns Hopkins University School of
    Medicine and Hospital
Baltimore, Maryland

Rajiv Shah, MD (Question 29)
Vitreo-Retinal Fellow
Retina Service
Wills Eye Institute
Philadelphia, Pennsylvania

Sana S. Siddique, MD (Questions 5 and 22)
Research Fellow
Massachusetts Eye Research & Surgery
    Institution
Cambridge, Massachusetts

Wendy M. Smith, MD (Question 46)
Clinical Fellow, Uveitis and Ocular
    Immunology
National Eye Institute
Bethesda, Maryland

Eric B. Suhler, MD, MPH (Question 24)
Chief of Ophthalmology
Portland VA Medical Center
Co-Director, Uveitis Clinic
Casey Eye Institute
Associate Professor of Ophthalmology
Oregon Health and Science University
Portland, Oregon

Sarah Syeda, BSc(MedSci) (Question 43)
University of Glasgow
Glasgow, United Kingdom

Joseph Tauber, MD (Question 12)
Tauber Eye Center
Kansas City, Missouri

*Simon Taylor, MA, PhD, FHEA, FRCOphth
    (Question 7)*
NIHR Clinical Lecturer in Ophthalmology
UCL Institute of Ophthalmology
London, United Kingdom
Acting Consultant Ophthalmic Surgeon
Royal Surrey County Hospital
Guildford, United Kingdom

Howard H. Tessler, MD (Question 32)
Professor of Ophthalmology
Department of Ophthalmology and Visual
    Sciences
University of Illinois at Chicago
Chicago, Illinois

Jennifer E. Thorne, MD, PhD (Question 33)
Chief, Division of Ocular Immunology
Associate Professor of Ophthalmology and
    Epidemiology
The Wilmer Eye Institute
Johns Hopkins School of Medicine
Baltimore, Maryland

Evangelia Tsironi, MD (Question 18)
Assistant Professor of Ophthalmology
University of Thessaly Medical School
Department of Ophthalmology
University Ophthalmology Clinic
Mezourlo, Larissa, Greece

Harvey Siy Uy, MD (Question 49)
Clinical Associate Professor of
    Ophthalmology
Sentro Oftalmologico Jose Rizal
University of the Philippines
Manila, Philippines
Director for Research
Asian Eye Institute
Makati, Philippines

Albert T. Vitale, MD (Question 48)
Professor Ophthalmology and Visual
    Sciences
Chief, Uveitis Division
Member, Vitreoretinal Division
John A. Moran Eye Center
University of Utah
Salt Lake City, Utah

Paul Yang, MD, PhD (Question 48)
John A. Moran Eye Center
University of Utah
Salt Lake City, Utah

Ellen N. Yu, MD (Question 43)
Institute of Ophthalmology
St. Luke's Medical Center
Quezon City, Philippines

Manfred Zierhut, MD, PhD (Question 13)
Professor of Ophthalmology
Centre of Ophthalmology
University of Tuebingen
Tuebingen, Germany

Introduction

Uveitis, the third leading cause of preventable blindness in developed countries, may occur as a consequence of trauma, infection, autoimmunity, or malignancy. Discerning the cause of the intraocular inflammation may take time and considerable work, with efforts akin to those of an internist trying to determine the cause of a patient's episodic fever and chronic fatigue. Such activity may not be especially appealing to doctors who have been attracted into the world of ophthalmology, with its microsurgical elegance and rapid gratification from refractive surgery or from cataract surgery. Many textbooks on the subject of uveitis and many learned publications in peer-reviewed literature have been published on the causes and treatments of patients with uveitis, and yet we, as uveitis specialists, continue to hear certain questions "on the curbside" repeatedly.

This monograph has been produced in an effort to help comprehensive ophthalmologists and other eye care specialists obtain a quick "consult" on just such questions. It is our collective hope that the answers to these 49 questions will prove to be helpful to those ophthalmologists who care for patients with uveitis in their practices and, additionally, that the questions and answers will also make clear that referral sooner rather than later to an ocular immunologist/uveitis specialist for co-management can be both intellectually fulfilling and sight saving for the patient.

C. Stephen Foster, MD, FACS, FACR
Clinical Professor of Ophthalmology, Harvard Medical School
President & CEO, Massachusetts Eye Research & Surgery Institution
Founder & President, Ocular Immunology & Uveitis Foundation
Cambridge, Massachusetts

ARE THERE STANDARD LABORATORY TESTS THAT NEED TO BE ORDERED IN A PATIENT WITH UVEITIS?

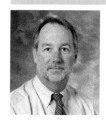

Neal P. Barney, MD

Uveitis laboratory testing should be tailored to each patient as there is no agreed upon standard set of tests to be performed. The tailored diagnostic work-up, including laboratory testing, is determined by the detailed history, thorough review of systems, clinical findings, and the differential diagnosis.

Uveitis is a leading cause of blindness worldwide. The majority of patients are managed by general ophthalmologists and do not require care from a uveitis specialist. Electing to perform laboratory testing may be guided by several principles. A specific diagnosis is not always possible or necessary for the management of uveitis. However, some uveitis entities (eg, Fuchs' heterochromic iridocyclitis, herpes zoster ophthalmicus, and serpiginous choroiditis) are diagnosed on clinical findings and do not need laboratory testing. It is important to keep in mind that there are few reliable systemic markers of ocular disease activity. Most commonly, diagnostic testing is performed based on frequency of recurrence. If the patient suffers easily treated, unilateral, nongranulomatous, and anterior uveitis, the second occurrence should be a reason for laboratory investigation. A positive review of systems with a constellation of findings suggestive of systemic disease that would account for the presence of uveitis should be evaluated by laboratory testing. Uveitis that is either granulomatous, intermediate in location, or presents as posterior uveitis with retinal vasculitis should undergo laboratory evaluation.

Once a decision is made to construct a tailored laboratory investigation, initial parsing begins with age, gender, geographic location of the patient, and anatomic location of the uveitis. A young man with abrupt onset of unilateral, recurrent pain, redness, and photophobia as anterior uveitis would be evaluated differently than a geriatric woman with the slow development of hazy vision in both eyes found to have vitritis. Uveitis patients in areas of high parasitic infection would have testing different from those in urban areas of developed countries. Finally, the list of differential diagnoses is paramount in constructing the list of tests to be performed.

As a list of tests is determined, priority is given to those tests with high specificity, high sensitivity, and low cost. Treponemal-based testing for syphilis is an example of a commonly performed test for all forms of uveitis. The test has high sensitivity and specificity. Moreover, syphilis is considered a great mimicker of various other uveitides; infection confers a positive response to testing for life, and syphilis is specifically treatable. Testing for a specific human leukocyte antigen subtype may prove useful when the history and exam point to certain uveitis syndromes.

Laboratory testing of uveitis patients is not limited to hematologic and serologic modalities. Noninvasive testing, such as radiographic evaluations, has a role when indicated. The finding of sacro-iliac joint narrowing would be important to the long-term general health of a young man who has no accompanying back pain but recurrent anterior uveitis. Invasive tests may be nonocular or ocular. Nonocular invasive testing may incur significant risks as in cerebrospinal fluid analysis or minimal risk as in tuberculosis skin testing. There are varying levels of risk associated with invasive ocular testing. While conjunctival biopsy looking for sarcoidosis may be accomplished with little risk, most recovery of intraocular tissues for examination has moderate risk. Obtaining aqueous, vitreous, or a retina-choroid biopsy may be performed in the setting of severe vision loss in one eye, with vision threat to the other or suspicion of a disease process that will threaten the general health of the patient. An advantage of obtaining ocular fluids or tissues is the specific testing that may be performed. Light, electron, and immunohistochemical microscopy may prove very revealing of specific disease entity. Such may be the case in primary central nervous system lymphoma with ocular involvement. Although the pathologic review may result in specific diagnosis, it is not uncommon to need to evaluate multiple specimens in the face of a high index of suspicion and negative findings on initial biopsy.

Ocular imaging has 2 roles in the evaluation of uveitis patients. Confirmation of anatomic changes that lead to vision loss is very important. If these changes are reversible, the use of therapy with significant risk of side effects is warranted. Improvement in the images obtained following therapy is also a role for documenting the appearance prior to treatment. Diagnostic imaging may uncover findings not readily seen on exam. Optic nerve head swelling and choroidal lesions may be uncovered when not suspected.

A specific list of laboratory tests is not recommended in uveitis patients. The selection of a tailored group of tests is determined by approaching the uveitis patient much the same as an internal medicine patient. The thorough history and complete review of systems coupled with a careful examination will allow the development of a differential diagnosis to guide diagnostic testing.

Suggested Readings

Foster CS, Vitale AT. *Diagnosis and Treatment of Uveitis.* Philadelphia, PA: Saunders; 2002.

Nussenblatt R, Whitcup SM. *Uveitis, Fundamentals and Clinical Practice: Expert Consult—Online and Print.* 4th ed. Oxford, UK: Elsevier; 2010.

What Is the Quality and Strength of Evidence in Peer-Reviewed Medical Literature on the Subject of Employment of Steroid-Sparing Immunomodulatory Therapy in the Care of Patients With Uveitis?

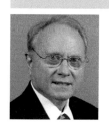

C. Stephen Foster, MD, FACS, FACR

The advent of corticosteroid use for the treatment of uveitis, as developed by Gordon and McLean[1] in 1950, revolutionized the care of patients with uveitis. While all drugs have potential side effects, some, including corticosteroids, are guaranteed to produce highly undesirable side effects if used for prolonged periods. Indeed, the development of cataract and glaucoma became obvious within 1 year of the introduction of corticosteroid therapy for treating uveitis. By the 1960s, thoughtful ophthalmologists were searching for nonsteroid substitutes to replace corticosteroids for their patients who had uveitis that relapsed with corticosteroid withdrawal. Wong and Hersh[2] introduced the idea of systemic methotrexate therapy for such patients, and many others subsequently published their experiences with other steroid-sparing immunomodulatory agents over the subsequent 40 years.[3-10]

The practice of evidence-based medicine relies upon data in peer-reviewed literature, which is judged to be high quality and strong evidence of efficacy and of substantial clinical benefit. The quality of the evidence can be judged based upon the sorts of studies and reports found in the peer-reviewed literature, with the highest quality evidence deemed to come from at least one well-designed, placebo-controlled, double-masked, randomized clinical trial. We in ophthalmology have suffered from lack of such trials because of the

Table 2-1

Literature Review Via the MEDLINE Database of English Language Reports From 1978 to 2003

Medication	*Strength and Quality of Evidence Recommending Use for Uevitis*
Methotrexate	Strong evidence, good quality
Azathioprine	Strong evidence, excellent quality (1 RCT#)
Mycophenolate	Strong evidence, good quality
Cyclosporine	Strong evidence, excellent quality (1 RCT#)
Tacrolimus	Weak evidence, good quality
Cyclophosphamide	Weak evidence, good quality (toxicity potential*)
Chlorambucil	Weak evidence, good quality (toxicity potential*)
Interferon alpha	Weak evidence, good quality

#RCT indicates randomized controlled trial.
*Toxicity potential results in downgraded evidence for employment for uveitis therapy.
Adapted from Okada AA. Immunomodulatory therapy for ocular inflammatory disease: a basic manual and review of the literature. *Ocul Immunol Inflamm.* 2005;13:335-351.

limited number of patients with specific types of uveitis or syndromes and the lack of sufficient financial support to conduct multicenter trials in uveitis therapy, thereby relegating us to depend upon evidence from cohort or case-controlled analytic studies, expert opinion panel consensus, and case series reports with common conclusions.

In 2003, I asked Dr. Annabelle Okada of the Department of Ophthalmology at Kyorin University School of Medicine in Tokyo, Japan, as a part of a program that I organized for an international meeting, to take on the task of reviewing the peer-reviewed literature on this subject. Her report on this matter[11] forms the core basis for this chapter. Her literature review via the MEDLINE database of English language reports from 1978 to 2003 led her to grade each report in the evidence-based scheme described previously (Table 2-1).

The American Uveitis Society also conducted a similar exercise, coming to the conclusion that there is very good evidence in peer-reviewed literature for both the safety and the efficacy of immunomodulatory therapy in the care of patients with various forms of ocular inflammatory disease, including uveitis.[12] Further, the panel of experts also opined that far too few ophthalmologists consider such therapy for their patients with steroid-dependent uveitis. This latter matter has been a central focus of the theme of each Uveitis Subspecialty Day at the annual meeting of the American Academy of Ophthalmology for the past 8 years as well.

Additionally, on the subject of safety of such therapy, several reports now document that a steroid-sparing approach is indeed safe, provided the prescribing physician is an expert in prescribing and monitoring these medications.[13,14] One topic of special concern through the years has been whether exposing patients with uveitis to immuno-modulatory agents increases their risk of dying or of developing a malignancy later in life. The aforementioned publications should give great comfort to all ophthalmologists who are caring for patients with steroid-dependent uveitis: there is no documentable evidence for such life-shortening complications in patients so treated.[14] The alkylating agents and the tumor necrosis factor inhibitor agents remain a concern in this sense, and thus we do not consider them first-line choices for steroid-sparing strategies.

References

1. Gordon DM, McLean JM. Effects of pituitary adrenocorticotropic hormone (ACTH) therapy in ophthalmologic conditions. *J Am Med Assoc.* 1950;142:1271-1276.
2. Wong VG, Hersh EM. Methotrexate in the therapy of cyclitis. *Trans Am Acad Ophthalmol Otolaryngol.* 1965;69:279-293.
3. Andrasch RH, Pirofsky B, Burns RP. Immunosuppressive therapy for severe chronic uveitis. *Arch Ophthalmol.* 1978;96:247-251.
4. Mamo JG, Azzam SA. Treatment of Behçet's disease with chlorambucil. *Arch Ophthalmol.* 1970;84:446-450.
5. Buckley CE III, Gills JP Jr. Cyclophosphamide therapy of peripheral uveitis. *Arch Intern Med.* 1969;124:29-35.
6. Newell FW, Krill AE, Thomson A. The treatment of uveitis with six-mercaptopurine. *Am J Ophthalmol.* 1966;61(5 Pt 2):1250-1255.
7. Michel SS, Ekong A, Baltatzis S, Foster CS. Multifocal choroiditis and panuveitis: immunomodulatory therapy. *Ophthalmology.* 2002;109:378-383.
8. Nussenblatt RB, Whitcup SM, de Smet MD, et al. Intraocular inflammatory disease (uveitis) and the use of oral tolerance: a status report. *Ann N Y Acad Sci.* 1996;778:325-337.
9. Benitez-del-Castillo JM, Martinez-de-la-Casa JM, Pato-Cour E, et al. Long-term treatment of refractory posterior uveitis with anti-TNF alpha (infliximab). *Eye (London).* 2005;19:841-845.
10. Yazici H, Pazarli H, Barnes CG, et al. A controlled trial of azathioprine in Behçet's syndrome. *N Engl J Med.* 1990;322:281-285.
11. Okada AA. Immunomodulatory therapy for ocular inflammatory disease: a basic manual and review of the literature. *Ocul Immunol Inflamm.* 2005;13:335-351.
12. Jabs DA, Rosenbaum JT, Foster CS, et al. Guidelines for the use of immunosuppressive drugs in patients with ocular inflammatory disorders: recommendations of an expert panel. *Am J Ophthalmol.* 2000;130:492-513.
13. Lane L, Tamesis R, Rodriguez A, et al. Systemic immunosuppressive therapy and the occurrence of malignancy in patients with ocular inflammatory disease. *Ophthalmology.* 1995;102:1530-1535.
14. Kempen J, Daniel E, Dunn JP, et al. Overall and cancer related mortality among patients with ocular inflammatory treated with immunosuppressive drugs: retrospective cohort study. *BMJ.* 2009;339:b2480.

QUESTION 3

WHEN SHOULD I REFER A PATIENT WITH UVEITIS TO A SPECIALIST?

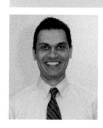

Yasir J. Sepah, MBBS
(co-authored with Quan Dong Nguyen, MD, MSc)

Uveitis is a major cause of vision loss in the developed world. Approximately 10% of the cases of reported vision loss worldwide may be attributed to uveitis. Economically, the United States alone spends more than $240 million annually on health care for patients with uveitis and its consequent morbidity. Often, uveitis patients may not be managed properly at the onset of the disease, and referral to a specialist is made only after the eye has suffered from irreversible damages. Hence, timely referral is of significant importance in the quest to reduce incidence of vision loss secondary to uveitis.

A comprehensive ophthalmologist is usually the first health care provider who comes in contact with patients suffering from uveitis and who performs the initial work-up. Identifying the etiology of uveitis or, in certain cases, the underlying disease that manifests as uveitis, can be challenging. For example, patients might present with an incomplete or unclear history, making it difficult to determine, at the time of presentation, the time course of the disease: acute or chronic. Similarly, the severity of the inflammation (pupillary synechiae, vitreous haze, among others) might make it difficult to perform a detailed ocular examination to plan for proper interventions.

Corticosteroids remain the only United States Food and Drug Administration (FDA) approved therapy for noninfectious uveitis. Although steroids are very effective in controlling inflammation initially, their long-term use is often associated with significant complications and side effects. The use of steroid-sparing agents is indicated if chronic steroid usage (7.5 mg or more of prednisone or equivalent daily) is required to control the inflammation. Immunomodulatory therapy (IMT; eg, antimetabolites, calcineurin inhibitors, alkylating agents, and biologics) is effective and appropriate, but its usage is also not without risks. Patients being treated with these agents require very thorough and experienced clinical oversight by specialists who are familiar with employing such classes of drugs.

In order to provide the best possible care to patients with uveitis, there are several key points and features that a comprehensive ophthalmologist should employ as a basis of referral to a uveitis specialist:

- *Goals of therapy:* Uveitis can be either acute or chronic in nature; both infectious and noninfectious uveitis can follow either of these courses. Nonetheless, the goals of therapy remain the same and include preservation of visual acuity, prompt identification of all sources of inflammation, zero tolerance toward any degree of inflammation, and proper management of complications (eg, macular edema, cataract, and glaucoma). If such goals cannot be achieved, the patients should be referred.

- *Etiology of uveitis:* Differentiation between infectious and noninfectious etiology cannot be overemphasized when uveitis is detected or suspected. Because corticosteroids are often the first-line therapy in the management of noninfectious uveitis, every effort should be made to rule out infectious etiology. Unfortunately, the etiology of inflammation cannot be ascertained in many cases. In such a scenario, empirical treatment with steroids may be warranted. However, even in such situations, a trial of systemic steroids should be considered prior to local administration due to the potentially sight-threatening consequences of treating infectious uveitis initially with local steroids. In order to avoid any undesirable consequences of therapy, in selected uveitic cases of uncertain etiology, or when the caring physician believes that he or she does not have the means to perform proper studies or procedures to make the diagnosis, the patients should be referred.

- *Nature of presentation:* The status of evaluation of the disease should always be kept in mind when managing patients with uveitis. If a patient presents for the first time with a mild case but bilateral involvement and has not been evaluated previously, the physician can consider initiating the work-up before making a referral to a specialist. On the other hand, if a patient has been previously evaluated and the work-up has been noninformative or the therapy has not been effective and the patient is now presenting with an exacerbation, then a referral is appropriate. Furthermore, it is important to remember that inadequate or unsatisfactory response to therapy may indicate that the etiology may not have been detected during the work-up. The patients should then be referred for a thorough evaluation.

- *Atypical presentation/masquerade syndromes:* Distinguishing among different etiologies of uveitis can be extremely challenging. It is not only important for an ophthalmologist to differentiate among causes but also to recognize atypical presentations. An illustrated example may be the multiple birdshot retinochoroidopathy-like lesions in a 40-year-old patient. In this case, one should be aware that birdshot retinochoroidopathy in general is a disease of the elderly, and one should therefore also consider other causes of such lesions in a relatively young patient. There are numerous conditions that can masquerade as uveitis but are managed quite differently. Thus, it is important that such masquerading syndromes are identified and managed properly. In the previously mentioned scenario, metastatic disease or primary ocular malignancy should be ruled out before starting the patient on any type of immunomodulatory therapy. When the presentation is "atypical," it is appropriate to refer the patients so proper evaluations and management can be executed.

- *Duration of disease:* Morbidity in eyes with uveitis is a result of chronic and recurrent episodes of inflammation, duration of each episode, frequency of attacks, and anatomic location of uveitis. Such repeated attacks may cause cumulative damage that could lead to irreversible tissue damage over time. In order to avoid cumulative damage of the disease, it is important that the disease is managed aggressively and any inflammation is eradicated as quickly as possible. There should be zero tolerance for any degree of inflammation. If the goal of complete control of inflammation is not achievable, the patients should be referred.

- *Choice of therapy:* Unfortunately, 28% to 59% of noninfectious uveitis patients will develop visual loss that requires a therapy beyond corticosteroids. Because of the numerous systemic and ocular complications associated with long-term use of steroids, it is not advisable to use corticosteroids for more than 6 months. When a patient is found to require a longer course of steroid therapy in order to fully control his or her disease, the patient should be referred to a uveitis specialist for discussion of other therapeutic options, including IMT and other steroid-sparing agents, sustained-release devices, or combination therapy.

Summary

Uveitis is a potentially sight-threatening condition of protean etiologies and is an important cause of ocular morbidity, including vision loss. The management of uveitis can be quite complex and can involve employment of multiple therapeutic options, some of which do have potential significant and serious side effects. Timely referral to uveitis specialists is of utmost priority and importance to allow correct diagnosis and prompt and aggressive treatment with appropriate therapeutic agents, which may help to preserve vision and reduce the risks of irreversible ocular injury secondary to cumulative damage in patients with uveitis.

Suggested Readings

Nguyen QD, Callanan D, Dugel P, Godfrey DG, Goldstein DA, Wilensky JT. Treating chronic noninfectious posterior segment uveitis: the impact of cumulative damage. Proceedings of an expert panel roundtable discussion. *Retina.* 2006;(Suppl):1-16.

Nguyen QD, Hatef E, Kayen B, et al. A cross-sectional study of the current treatment patterns in noninfectious uveitis among specialists in the United States. *Ophthalmology.* 2011;118:184-190. Epub 2010 Aug 3.

ARE THERE SPECIAL CONSIDERATIONS IN TREATING A CHILD WITH UVEITIS?

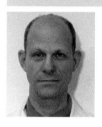

Ron Neumann, MD

Treating a Child Translates to Treating the Whole Family Unit

Treating the uveitic child includes caring for the child and his or her family unit simultaneously. Trusting relationships with the family are vital to create a comfort zone for the child, striving for compliance and collaboration with the team that is critical for a successful therapeutic process.

The family commonly presents with intense anxiety and sometimes with inaccurate information derived from the Internet. Typically, the parents are worrying about the implications of the disease on the entirety of the child's life.

Fears commonly exceed reality. Taking the time once in the beginning of the therapeutic process to sit with the family outside of the busy clinic hours, setting their expectations, telling the story of the disease—being realistic and yet comforting, and posing hope where hope is due—would be rewarding in the long run. This would also be a perfect opportunity to set the importance of therapy and compliant follow-up.

The Classic Juvenile Syndromes

Juvenile idiopathic arthritis (JIA)-associated uveitis, whether involving joints (as in most cases) or not, is most common in children. This syndrome may appear very early—2 years old and up, with younger children tending to develop more severe disease. Early diagnosis requires close follow-up of all children diagnosed with JIA regardless of ocular complaints. The disease is relentlessly chronic but sometimes may lose its punch following adolescence. The inflammation is focused to the anterior chamber and, left untreated, may result in grave damage. It is not the scope of this short chapter to detail JIA, and I would refer the reader to the book by Foster and Vitale for further reading.[1] Suffice to say here that the complexity and the grave prognosis of this syndrome, if left untreated or partially treated, has led to the concept of "zero" tolerance for anterior chamber inflammation. The other syndrome commonly seen in young adults is pars planitis, typified with inflammation of the vitreous body and the peripheral retinal vitreous junction. Pars planitis ranges from a mild disease that may warrant follow-up only to a highly destructive entity that threatens retinal integrity and hence vision.

The Symptoms, Their Significance, and the Significance of Their Absence

VISUAL ACUITY

The younger the child is, the less aware he or she is of visual acuity loss, especially when only one eye is involved. It is, therefore, impractical for parents and caregivers to rely on toddlers' and young elementary school children's complaints. Careful examination of visual acuity in each visit is therefore warranted.

REDNESS

Unlike classic acute uveitis syndromes where redness is often an integral part of the inflammatory picture, JIA uveitis and pars planitis usually do not cause ocular redness. For this reason, redness is not reliable in the follow-up of uveitis in childhood, and each evaluation requires a meticulous slit-lamp examination.

PAIN

Unlike classic uveitis entities in adults, JIA uveitis usually does not result in pain even when inflammation increases. Adults carrying the disease from childhood often report "unease" when their inflammations intensify. Similarly, pars planitis only rarely causes severe pain, and the symptoms reported by patients usually relate to visual disturbances.

OCULAR SECRETIONS AND TEARING

These are not part of the uveitis picture, although patients often worry that incidental tearing or secretions signify increase of their disease activity.

Thus, the classic complaints that help us follow adults with uveitis and sometimes distinguish real emergency from trivial complaints are useless in children. Following children with uveitis necessitates frequent slit-lamp examinations, and one can hardly rely on patients' complaints and reports.

Amblyopia and the Treating Team

Optical axis opacities (cataracts, band shape keratopathy) in toddlers and young children may cause permanent loss of vision due to quick progression of occlusion amblyopia. This may often dictate advancement of surgical treatments aimed to clear the optical axis combined with optometric correction and amblyopia therapy. Thus, a team consisting of ocular inflammation, ocular pediatric, surgical, optometric, pediatric rheumatologist, and psychological experts is necessary to offer adequate medical care for these patients.

Corticosteroids and Immunosuppression in Children

All known corticosteroid complications in adults may manifest in childhood too. Growth retardation is relevant in children prior to bone growth center closure. Increased psychomotor activity may greatly reduce kids' performance in school. Cushingoid changes are most notable in kids and, along with weight gain, are disfiguring and severely affect children's social status. In addition, hirsutism, striae, osteopenia, and even osteoporosis leading to fractures, hypertension, and diabetes may all manifest in childhood. I find that tolerability in childhood is much reduced compared to adults and steroid-sparing agents should be considered early on. Topically applied corticosteroids in children should be restricted as much as possible, fearing cataracts that may quickly lead to amblyopia. Aspiration to completely eradicate all anterior chamber inflammatory cells frequently conflicts with the unavoidable cataract and high risk of glaucoma inherent to steroid therapy. Fluorometholone, rimexolone, and loteprednol (Lotemax) with less propensity for intraocular pressure (IOP) elevation may be helpful in milder cases. This is one of the many reasons for the early move to steroid-sparing immunosuppressive strategies in children.

Methotrexate and azathioprine (Imuran) are nicely tolerated by children. Similar to adults, frequent blood counts and liver function tests are mandatory. The main limiting adverse event in children treated with methotrexate is nausea. This appears to be significant in approximately half of the patients and may result in vomiting and ultimately treatment failure. Injecting methotrexate intramuscularly or subcutaneously may provide some relief from the nausea; otherwise, azathioprine or mycophenolate mofetil may provide a similar therapeutic effect. Failing this line of anti-metabolites, one can resort to tumor necrosis factor-alpha inhibitors, specifically infliximab and adalimumab. Etanercept should not be used for uveitis.

Glaucoma

Glaucoma is probably the most severe complication that is potentially blinding in the context of uveitis in children. Approximately 40% of the children with JIA uveitis develop glaucoma,[2] and it is considered to be one of the most common complications or even the most common complication of JIA uveitis.[3] More concerning is the fact that glaucoma in children with JIA tends to be more difficult than in adults, leading to twice the number of glaucoma surgeries in children.[4] It is critical to spare no efforts in pursuing target pressure and refer relatively quickly to surgery when target pressure is not obtained and damage starts to develop. It is critically important to quiet inflammation first before taking the patient to surgery, even if this means delay with uncontrolled IOP.

References

1. Foster CS, Vitale AT, eds. *Diagnosis and Treatment of Uveitis.* Philadelphia, PA: WB Saunders; 2001.
2. Sijssens KM, Rothova A, Berendschot TT, de Boer JH. Ocular hypertension and secondary glaucoma in children with uveitis. *Ophthalmology.* 2006;113:853-859, e2.
3. Holland GN, Denove CS, Yu F. Chronic anterior uveitis in children: clinical characteristics and complications. *Am J Ophthalmol.* 2009;147:667-678, e5. Epub 2009 Feb 4.
4. Heinz C, Koch JM, Zurek-Imhoff B, Heiligenhaus A. Prevalence of uveitic secondary glaucoma and success of nonsurgical treatment in adults and children in a tertiary referral center. *Ocul Immunol Inflamm.* 2009;17: 243-248.

HOW SHOULD I TREAT A PATIENT WITH UVEITIS AND DIABETES MELLITUS?

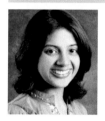

Sana S. Siddique, MD

An association between diabetes and anterior uveitis suggesting an immunological cause was first proposed by Guy and associates in 1984.[1] Soon after, in 1988, Rothova and associates reported that 20 of 340 patients with anterior uveitis (6%) suffered from diabetes mellitus.[2] They found that 63% (16) of diabetic patients with idiopathic uveitis had type I diabetes mellitus. Furthermore, 75% (12) of them suffered from severe diabetic complications, including angiopathy, nephropathy, and neuropathy. All of the diabetic patients with idiopathic uveitis were first diagnosed with diabetes mellitus.[2]

The association between diabetes mellitus and ocular disease might be explained by the damage that chronic hyperglycemia exerts on the microvasculature. While this damage may not be readily noticeable in other organs of the body, the eye is particularly sensitive to these changes. Once the blood vessels in the eye are affected, they produce myriad eye diseases, including ocular inflammation and uveitis.

Patients with diabetes mellitus who experience a first episode of uveitis usually present with decreased vision and severe anterior uveitis that might require more aggressive anti-inflammatory therapy than patients with uveitis not associated with diabetes.[3] The aim of uveitis therapy in patients with diabetes is dual: first, to prevent visual loss, to improve symptoms, and to decrease ocular morbidity; second, to achieve glycemic control by closely monitoring glucose levels, blood pressure, and renal function. Levels of hemoglobin-A1C are of utmost importance in assessing the patient's glycemic control over time.

The first step in the treatment of uveitis in patients with diabetes is the aggressive use of topical corticosteroids to rapidly extinguish inflammation. The corticosteroids should be discontinued in a tapering manner to prevent rebound inflammation.

In cases of refractory uveitis, the use of regional or even intraocular corticosteroids, as well as systemic corticosteroid therapy, particularly in a patient with diabetes mellitus, is acceptable unless a contraindication exists. Keep in mind that the aim is not only to get the inflammation under control but also to maintain glucose levels within normal limits. If glycemic control is not achieved while on systemic corticosteroids, it is imperative to use insulin to decrease the blood glucose levels and prevent ketoacidosis. In such instances, close collaboration with the primary care physician and/or endocrinologist is paramount.

The use of systemic corticosteroids in patients with diabetes must be judicious. It is well known that these have a potent diabetogenic effect by upregulating key regulatory enzymes in the liver that promote gluconeogenesis. Moreover, steroids also decrease insulin release from the pancreas and increase its peripheral resistance. Such effects are secondary to the inhibition of the expression of a specific glucose transporter (GLUT-4) in the skeletal and adipose tissue. These complex metabolic effects of corticosteroids elevate postprandial and fasting glucose. In addition, steroids also elevate blood pressure. Hence, the use of systemic corticosteroids must be cautious, and regular monitoring of blood pressure, renal function, and blood glucose levels is mandatory. It is important to emphasize that systemic corticosteroids should not be used for a prolonged period, and a determined effort must be made to taper the steroids, with initiation of immunomodulatory therapy (IMT) in the quest for steroid-free durable remission of sight-threatening uveitis. That said, an occasion may arise in which sight-threatening uveitis in a patient with diabetes mellitus calls for urgent but brief use of systemic corticosteroids.

The step ladder approach in steroid-sparing immunomodulatory therapy must be tailored to each patient, depending on the severity and underlying associated systemic disease. When prescribing IMT, it is important to keep in mind the effects of therapy on the blood glucose levels, renal and hepatic function, and blood pressure. Additionally, IMT has the potential to decrease the circulating white blood cells, increasing the risk of infection. Thus, monitoring with a complete blood count, renal and hepatic function tests, along with blood pressure and blood glucose levels every 6 weeks is imperative (Table 5-1).

At the Massachusetts Eye Research and Surgery Institution, we generally employ agents within the anti-metabolite group initially: methotrexate, mycophenolate mofetil, and azathioprine. Cyclosporine A (CsA), a calcineurin inhibitor, might be used in combination or as monotherapy in patients who do not tolerate anti-metabolite agents. It is important to note that CsA has a diabetogenic effect due to its effects on postprandial carbohydrate metabolism and interferes with the action of oral hypoglycemic drugs, such as tolbutamide and glyburide.[4] However, CsA does not interfere with the actions of neutral protamine Hagedorn insulin. Special attention must be given to cyclosporine adverse effects that include nephropathy, hyperlipidemia, and secondary hypertension, particularly in patients with metabolic syndrome. The use of alkylating agents such as chlorambucil and cyclophosphamide is usually reserved for vision-threatening uveitis or life-threatening vasculitis; we recommend the use of intravenous cyclophosphamide and postmedication fluids to reduce the risk of bladder carcinoma. The use of biologic response modifiers, either subcutaneous or intravenous, is reserved for patients who are intolerant to oral therapy, who cannot take oral medications, or who are refractory to first-line therapy. This step ladder approach is deferred to the "best drug" selection if an associated systemic disease is

Table 5-1
Side Effects of Immunosuppressants

Immunosuppressant	Important Side Effects in Diabetics	Monitoring Q6 Weeks
Methotrexate	Hyperglycemia, hepatotoxicity, renal toxicity, infection	CBC, LFT, RFT, casual blood glucose
Azathioprine	Myelosuppression, hepatotoxicity	CBC, LFT
Mycophenolate Mofetil	Myelosuppression, hepatotoxicity	CBC, LFT
Cyclophosphamide	Myelosuppression	CBC
Chlorambucil	Myelosuppression	CBC
Infliximab, Etanercept	Cytopenia	WBC
Adalimumab	Cytopenia, hyperglycemia, hypertension	WBC, casual blood glucose, blood pressure

LFT indicates liver function tests; RFT, renal function tests; CBC, complete blood count; WBC, white blood cells.

identified; the drug that most effectively controls the uveitis associated with that particular disease is chosen, and, in such instances, working closely with the primary care physician and/or endocrinologists is essential.

The safest approach in uveitis therapy for a diabetic is to use medication that has minimal effects on blood glucose levels and renal and liver function. Azathioprine, mycophenolate mofetil, and the alkylating agents are a safe choice, but, nevertheless, close monitoring must be implemented.

References

1. Guy RJ, Richards F, Edmonds ME, Watkins PJ. Diabetic autonomic neuropathy and iritis: an association suggesting an immunological cause. *Br Med J (Clin Res Ed).* 1984;289:343-345.
2. Rothova A, Meenken C, Michels RP, Kijlstra A. Uveitis and diabetes mellitus. *Am J Ophthalmol.* 1988;106:17-20.
3. Oswal KS, Sivaraj RR, Stavrou P, Murray PI. Clinical features of patients with diabetes mellitus presenting with their first episode of uveitis. *Ocul Immunol Inflamm.* 2009;17:390-393.
4. Pollock SH, Reichbaum MI, Collier BH, D'Souza MJ. Inhibitory effect of cyclosporine A on the activity of oral hypoglycemic agents in rats. *J Pharmacol Exp Ther.* 1991;258:8-12.

WHAT UNDERLYING CAUSES SHOULD BE FOREMOST IN THE DIFFERENTIAL DIAGNOSIS OF ACUTE HYPERTENSIVE UVEITIS?

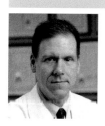

Russell W. Read, MD, PhD

The development of acute anterior uveitis is usually associated with a lowering of intraocular pressure, as inflammation of the ciliary body results in a decrease in aqueous production while aqueous outflow is enhanced by increased uveoscleral outflow. When faced with a case of acute anterior uveitis with increased intraocular pressure, the ophthalmologist must consider several possibilities. I prefer to begin thinking broadly, narrowing down the possibilities with the pertinent positives and negatives of the details of the existing case. The mechanisms by which intraocular pressure can be elevated include 2 possibilities: 1) an increase in aqueous inflow, or 2) a decrease in aqueous outflow. I am unaware of uveitic diseases that result in an increase in aqueous production, so all relevant causes to be considered focus on impaired outflow. Consideration of this clinical scenario is well suited to an algorithmic approach, presented via outline form to follow. Determining the presence or absence of each of the possibilities presented is relatively straightforward using standard ophthalmologic examination techniques, including slit-lamp biomicroscopy, gonioscopy, and dilated fundus examination.

Mechanisms of Decreased Outflow

I. Inhibition of access to trabecular meshwork (TM)
  A. Angle closure
    1. Peripheral anterior synechiae (PAS)

a) The patient with "acute hypertensive uveitis" may in fact have chronic disease with a current exacerbation and long-standing development of PAS that suddenly reaches the point of complete angle closure.

b) Disease entities to consider:

   (1) Any acute recurrent or chronic uveitis involving the anterior segment may produce PAS. The status of the angle, especially in the setting of continued active disease, should be monitored with regular gonioscopy.

   (2) The human leukocyte antigen (HLA)-B27-associated entities, with their frequent presence of fibrin in the anterior chamber, are particularly likely to result in synechiae.

2. Iris bombé secondary to pupillary seclusion

   a) As above, repeated attacks of anterior uveitis can eventually result in 360 degrees of posterior synechiae with peripheral iris bowing sufficient to occlude the angle.

3. Neovascularization of the iris and angle

   a) Neovascularization due to uveitis alone is uncommon. However, uveitis affecting the posterior segment could result in retinal ischemia with resultant increased vascular endothelial growth factor (VEGF) production.

   b) Disease entities to consider:

   (1) Occlusive vasculitis (viral retinitis, Behçet's disease, sarcoid, systemic lupus erythematosus, antineutrophil cytoplasmic antibody-associated vasculitis).

   (2) Inflammatory lesions compressing the optic nerve and causing vein occlusion, such as sarcoid.

4. Anterior rotation of the lens-iris diaphragm

   a) Uveitis affecting the posterior segment and producing choroidal thickening, serous effusions, or scleral edema (such as in scleritis) can produce anterior rotation of the lens-iris diaphragm, including the ciliary body, resulting in angle closure.

   (1) Disease entities to consider:

       (a) Vogt-Koyanagi-Harada disease

       (b) Sympathetic ophthalmia

       (c) Posterior scleritis

B. Clogging of TM by cells or debris

   1. Lens-induced uveitis

   a) Disease entities to consider:

   (1) Phacolytic uveitis

       (a) A hypermature lens, leaking lens proteins through its capsule, stimulates a macrophage infiltration with phagocytosis of that lens material and clogging of the TM by those macrophages.

   (2) Phacoantigenic uveitis

       (a) Disruption of the lens capsule incites a granulomatous inflammatory reaction that may also clog the TM.

   2. Chronic retinal detachment (Schwartz syndrome)

   a) The presence of a rhegmatogenous retinal detachment, typically long-standing, may result in release of photoreceptor outer segments that exit the subretinal space through the retinal break to eventually reach the TM and produce increased intraocular pressure.

II. Outflow resistance within the trabecular meshwork
  A. Trabeculitis
    1. Disease entities to consider:
      a) Herpetic
        (1) Herpes simplex
        (2) Herpes zoster
        (3) Cytomegalovirus (CMV)
        (4) All of these are typically unilateral. Herpes simplex and zoster uveitis will frequently result in transillumination defects of the iris that are either broad (in the case of zoster) or patchy (in the case of simplex). CMV uveitis is difficult to diagnosis by clinical characteristics alone. Aqueous humor aspiration for polymerase chain reaction may be helpful in confirming the diagnosis.
      b) Toxoplasmosis
      c) Miscellaneous, possibly infectious
        (1) Fuch's heterochromic iridocyclitis
        (2) Posner-Schlossman syndrome
        (3) Each of these has been linked to herpetic disease, but a definitive etiological connection is lacking.
  B. Corticosteroid response
    1. Any patient receiving topical, periocular, intraocular, or systemic corticosteroids for uveitis may develop elevated intraocular pressure.
      a) Typically delayed in onset
  C. Increased episcleral venous pressure
    1. Disease entities to consider
      a) Scleritis

Summary

While a number of different entities may result in elevation of the intraocular pressure in the setting of uveitis, this remains the exception to the rule. Infectious causes are particularly common if the angle is open. Careful history and examination will usually produce the diagnosis.

WHAT UNDERLYING CAUSES SHOULD BE FOREMOST IN THE DIFFERENTIAL DIAGNOSIS OF ACUTE HYPOPYON UVEITIS?

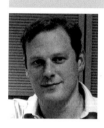

Simon Taylor, MA, PhD, FHEA, FRCOphth
(co-authored with Sue Lightman, PhD, FRCP, FRCOphth)

Acute hypopyon uveitis is uncommon and is characterized by the occurrence of a fluid level of cells in the anterior chamber. Hypopyons are most commonly white, but can occasionally be other colors, such as pink, brown, or black. Their presence reflects severe intraocular inflammation and can be associated with immune-mediated inflammation, infection, or malignancy. They can also occur secondary to microbial keratitis. A detailed history is mandatory, as is meticulous examination of the eye, as these will enable emergency management to be instituted in advance of the results of other investigations.

What Disorders Cause Hypopyon?

Hypopyon uveitis occurs in about 7% of patients with acute anterior uveitis, especially recurrent disease associated with human leukocyte antigen (HLA)-B27 positivity.[1,2] In patients with posterior uveitis, the most common association is Behçet's disease—6% of these patients develop hypopyon uveitis. In both of these, the inflammation is usually intense, and the patient is very symptomatic.

In patients who have recently had either cataract surgery or another intraocular procedure, including intravitreal therapy, the presence of a hypopyon is indicative of severe intraocular infection (Figure 7-1). This may occur in the first week following the procedure (acute endophthalmitis) or be delayed several weeks (chronic endophthalmitis). Worsening of chronic endophthalmitis can also occur following YAG capsulotomy, as previously localized infection is disseminated throughout the eye.

Figure 7-1. Hypopyon occurring in an eye with bacterial endophthalmitis occurring 4 days after cataract surgery.

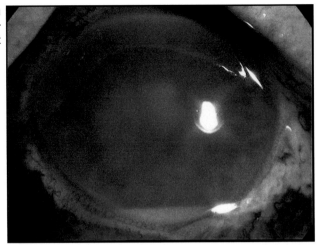

Figure 7-2. Hypopyon with iris infiltrates in a patient with lymphoma.

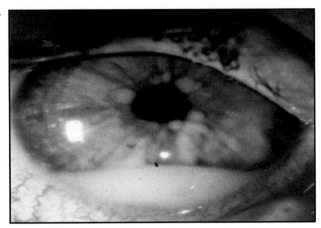

Intraocular toxocara infection can present with a hypopyon, usually in a white eye, but there may also be classic signs of a white retinal mass on fundal examination or signs of infection/inflammation throughout the eye. In patients who have been or who are systemically unwell with sepsis, endogenous endophthalmitis must be considered. This can present as unilateral or bilateral endophthalmitis with hypopyon, and the septic focus can be anywhere, including chest, skin, liver, and heart.[3] In patients who have had long lines for intravenous therapy, systemic candidiasis can occur. Ocular involvement with hypopyon uveitis can occur up to 2 weeks postinfection, and, therefore, the patient may present with a hypopyon uveitis after he or she has been discharged from the hospital.

In patients with a known history of malignancy, hypopyon uveitis is most likely to be related to this and occurs in leukemia, lymphoma (B- and T-cell types; Figure 7-2), and melanoma, as well as in other malignancies.[2] The eye may be white, and there may be a mass or masses visible on the iris. Retinoblastoma may present with a white eye and a hypopyon (Figure 7-3) and may thus mimic the signs seen in toxocara infection on clinical examination. A positive family history may help with the diagnosis.

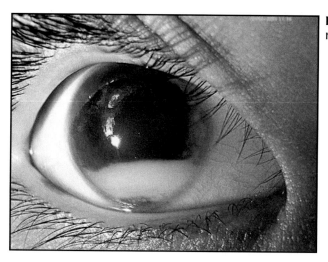

Figure 7-3. Hypopyon in a child with retinoblastoma.

Drugs such as rifabutin are known to be associated with hypopyon uveitis when given in association with clarithromycin and/or fluconazole.[2] Intraocular triamcinolone injection can result in a white hypopyon, and this can be due to the drug itself, secondary infective endophthalmitis, or as a result of sterile endophthalmitis.

What Questions Should You Ask?

Asking the correct questions is crucial at presentation and is aimed at distinguishing the above causes to narrow down the differential diagnosis. Some causes need to be identified immediately and treated as an emergency, such as hypopyon uveitis associated with exogenous or endogenous infection and acute anterior uveitis/panuveitis.[1,2,4] Hypopyon associated with malignancy may need emergency management if the intraocular pressure is high, such as occurs when the angle has been infiltrated, but usually can be investigated over the next few days.

Key questions include asking about previous episodes, HLA-B27 positivity or spondyloarthopathy, symptoms of Behçet's disease, recent relevant ocular procedures, recent systemic illness with a fever or hospital admission, diagnosis or treatment of malignant disease, and concurrent drug therapy.[3] Patients may not necessarily have associated any of these events or diagnoses with an eye problem, so they may not volunteer this information without direct questioning.

What Signs Should You Look For?

Most commonly, eyes with hypopyon uveitis are red eyes—those that require urgent management are nearly always red, with the exception that hypopyon uveitis occurring in Behçet's disease can sometimes occur in a white eye. In patients who are very photophobic, examination of the back of the eye may not be possible at the first visit, and in those with endophthalmitis, particularly when associated with bacterial infection, severe vitritis may impede an adequate fundal view. In both infective and inflammatory causes, fibrin and cells in the anterior chamber usually accompany the hypopyon, and it is paramount not to miss intraocular infection as the cause: infection must be considered in every patient with this clinical appearance, as injection of intraocular antibiotics may save the eye. White infiltrates on the iris may occur in patients with leukemia and lymphoma. White masses within the eye may occur with toxocara infection and retinoblastoma; ultrasound investigation may help to differentiate these, as calcium deposition can be seen in retinoblastoma.

References

1. Zaidi AA, Ying GS, Daniel E, et al. Hypopyon in patients with uveitis. *Ophthalmology.* 2010;117:366-372.
2. Ramsay A, Lightman S. Hypopyon uveitis. *Surv Ophthalmol.* 2001;46:1-18.
3. Jackson TL, Eykyn SJ, Graham EM, Stanford MR. Endogenous bacterial endophthalmitis: a 17-year prospective series and review of 267 reported cases. *Surv Ophthalmol.* 2003;48:403-423.
4. Sanghvi C, Mercieca K, Jones NP. Very severe HLA B27-associated panuveitis mimicking endophthalmitis: a case series. *Ocul Immunol Inflamm.* 2010;18:139-141.

WHEN SHOULD I CONSIDER USING SYSTEMIC CORTICOSTEROIDS TO TREAT UVEITIS?

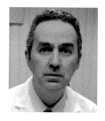

Alejandro Rodríguez-García, MD

Systemic corticosteroids, with immunosuppressive drugs when indicated, are the mainstay therapy for many forms of severe noninfectious intermediate, posterior, and panuveitis.[1]

Systemic prednisone has also been used to treat uveitis refractory to local therapy and to avoid undesirable side effects from topical medications, like increased intraocular pressure.[2]

During an acute attack of severe intraocular inflammation, systemic prednisone undoubtedly has the most effective and rapid response profile compared to any other kind of anti-inflammatory medication. Therefore, in patients with ocular inflammatory diseases, such as Vogt-Koyanagi-Harada (VKH) syndrome, sympathetic ophthalmia, optic neuritis, sarcoidosis, primary retinal vasculitis, and systemic vasculitis with ocular involvement (lupus erythematosus, polyarteritis nodosa, Wegener's granulomatosis) among others, the use of systemic prednisone during the acute phase is crucial to control the inflammatory response rapidly and to avoid ocular complications and sequelae derived from the uveitis (Figures 8-1 and 8-2).[3]

High-dose methyl-prednisolone intravenous pulse therapy is also recommended as initial therapy, followed by oral administration in patients with severe and/or uncontrolled ocular inflammation. I particularly recommend the administration of 750 to 1000 mg methyl-prednisolone IV pulses/day for 3 days for patients in the acute stage of VKH syndrome, patients with sympathetic ophthalmia, and those with acute optic neuritis, particularly in those suspicious for multiple sclerosis. In such cases, patients may need to be hospitalized and closely monitored with blood glucose levels, blood pressure, and the administration of an H2 blocker to avoid peptic ulcer disease.

Figure 8-1. Fluorescein angiogram of a patient showing the acute phase of VKH syndrome who was hospitalized and treated with intravenous methyl-prednisolone (1 g/day for 3 days) and continued on oral prednisone at 1 mg/kg/day for the following 3 weeks before tapering to less than 10 mg/day with excellent therapeutic response.

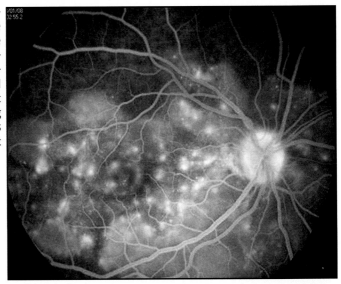

Figure 8-2. Late phase fluorescein angiogram of the left eye with acute VKH syndrome, showing extensive dye leakage from the serous retinal detachment on the posterior pole (same patient as in Figure 8-1) .

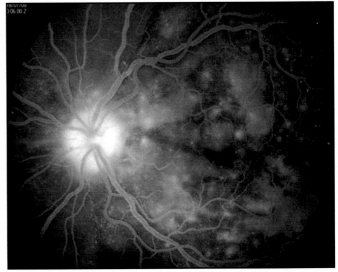

Oral corticosteroids are also frequently administered as prophylaxis for patients with uveitis at the time of cataract surgery.[4] In this respect, I advise patients to start or readjust oral prednisone 3 days before surgery to a dose of 40 to 60 mg/day and to continue so for 1 week after cataract removal and then taper it slowly according to the inflammatory status.

In some forms of infectious uveitis like severe ocular toxoplasmosis, herpetic uveitis, and neuro-syphilis, among others, systemic prednisone also plays a very important role as adjunctive therapy to control severe inflammation once the patient is on antibiotics for at least 3 days prior to corticosteroid administration (Figure 8-3).[5]

Patients in whom systemic corticosteroids should be avoided are those already overweight and patients with diabetes mellitus, hypercholesterolemia, arterial hypertension, coronary insufficiency, peptic ulcer, pregnancy, and also children under 16 years of age.

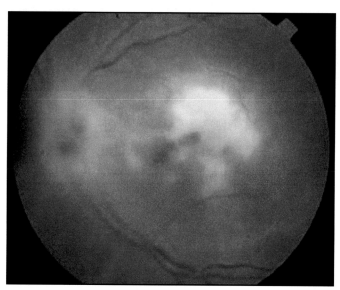

Figure 8-3. *Toxoplasma gondii* neuroretinitis with macular involvement in the left eye in a patient who needs to be treated with oral prednisone (1 mg/kg/day) along with systemic anti-*Toxoplasma* antibiotics.

The ideal administration for oral prednisone is in a single dose given in the morning. This is more physiologic because the natural peak of adrenal corticosteroid production occurs at this time. It also helps to reduce insomnia. The starting dose should be 1 to 1.5 mg/kg/day until a good control of inflammation is achieved, and then taper it down over a period of 4 to 6 weeks to a total dose of 10 mg/day or less and gradually reduce it until discontinuation.[1] Whenever a higher dose of corticosteroid therapy extends beyond this period of time, I strongly recommend giving all patients supplemental calcium (1.0 to 1.5 g/day) along with vitamin D (400 to 800 IU/day) to retard bone loss, and I encourage them to stop smoking, do weight-bearing exercises, and get regular dual-energy x-ray absorptiometry (DEXA) scans. Biphosphonates are also recommended for patients at higher risk of osteoporosis, including postmenopausal women without estrogen replacement therapy. I also recommend that all patients, particularly those with gastroesophageal reflux and those prone to develop peptic ulcer disease, should be put on an H2 blocker (eg, oral ranitidine 150 mg twice daily) or a proton pump inhibitor (eg, oral omeprazol, 20 mg/day). Sodium intake may need to be reduced, and potassium supplements may be necessary as well.

Baseline evaluation of patients on prolonged treatment with oral prednisone should include measuring the blood pressure, serum glucose, lipids (cholesterol and triglycerides), and electrolytes, particularly sodium and potassium levels. Patients at higher risk of developing osteoporosis should also have a bone densitometry every year. Finally, purified protein derivative (PPD) and HIV tests should also be considered in suspicious cases.[2]

With systemic corticosteroids, the expected therapeutic efficacy always has to be weighed against potential adverse effects. We need to remember that, even when used in the short term, systemic corticosteroids can lead to a number of adverse effects, including increased appetite, weight gain, Cushingoid appearance, gastrointestinal irritation and peptic ulceration, osteoporosis, pathologic fractures, muscular wasting, mental disturbances (eg, insomnia, psychosis, depression, and euphoria), sodium retention, potassium loss, arterial hypertension, diabetes mellitus, and adrenal insufficiency, among others. Alternate day dosing has previously been shown to be an effective strategy to reduce the side effects while maintaining the same corticosteroid effect.[2,3]

Summary

Systemic corticosteroids are necessary to treat acute episodes of intraocular inflammation related to severe noninfectious uveitis. It should be considered that doses greater than 5 mg/day for prolonged periods of time is undesirable; adjunctive immunosuppressive or biologic therapy is recommended in such situations in order to avoid serious and irreversible side effects.

References

1. Jabs DA, Rosenbaum JT, Foster JS, et al. Guidelines for the use of immunosuppressive drugs in patients with ocular inflammatory disorders: recommendations of an expert panel. *Am J Ophthalmol.* 2000;130:492-513.
2. Rothova A. Corticosteroids in uveitis. *Ophthalmol Clin N Am.* 2002;15:389-394.
3. Djalilian AR, Nussenblatt RB. Immunosuppression in uveitis. *Ophthalmol Clin N Am.* 2002;15:395-404.
4. Jancevski M, Foster CS. Cataracts and uveitis. *Curr Opin Ophthalmol.* 2010;21:10-14.
5. Engstrom RE Jr, Holland GN, Nussenblatt RB, Jabs DA. Current practices in the management of ocular toxoplasmosis. *Am J Ophthalmol.* 1991;111:601-610.

WHAT IS THE SINGLE MOST IMPORTANT SOURCE OF DIAGNOSTIC LEADS FOR UNCOVERING A DIAGNOSABLE CAUSE OF UVEITIS?

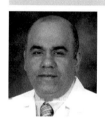

Amro Ali, MD
(co-authored with James T. Rosenbaum, MD)

After her annual check-up, a friend recently complained to us about her internist: "He talked to me a long time, but he did not even do a physical exam."

The internist may have missed the opportunity for a "laying on of hands," but at least he knew that the majority of all diagnoses in the practice of internal medicine are made or suspected by the medical history. We think that the same applies to ophthalmology, even if the specialty relies heavily on seeing the pathology.

Differential diagnosis rests on a 3-legged stool: history, exam, and laboratory testing. Uveitis falls into subsets based on etiology. Subsets are also defined by parameters that include anatomic location, symmetry (unilateral or bilateral), onset (insidious or sudden), continuity (continuous or episodic), duration (brief or persistent), and association with complications like posterior synechiae and glaucoma. While some of these variables require an ophthalmic examination (patients cannot tell you their intraocular pressure accurately without a measurement), patients do know if the disease is in one or both eyes, if the inflammation has had quiescent periods without therapy, and whether the disease began suddenly or over time. Moreover, the anatomic location can usually be surmised by the history. Pain, redness, and photophobia usually indicate the sudden onset of anterior inflammation. Glare generally means a cataract has formed. Floaters correlate well with cells and organization in the vitreous humor. If a patient has an associated systemic disease (eg, a history of chronic, inflammatory low back pain, painful oral ulcers, or frequent loose stools), that critical information will only be obtained by taking a history.

Taking a history begins with asking an open-ended question about the purpose of the visit. It continues with ascertaining the details related to the problem, such as when it began or what medications have been helpful. The past medical history, family history, and social history may each help to focus the differential diagnosis. For example, inflammatory lower back is related to human leukocyte antigen (HLA) B27 and is often common among multiple family members. Finally, a thorough review of systems is essential. Details related to joint, skin, bowel, lung, and central nervous system disease (as examples) might help clarify the nature of an ocular problem.

Of course, there are diseases that require an ophthalmic examination for diagnoses (eg, all the white dot syndromes like birdshot chorioretinopathy). There are also diseases for which the physical examination might not be pathognomonic, but the physical finding nonetheless reveals more than the history; examples include the subretinal infiltrates of ocular lymphoma or the macular star of cat scratch fever. However, these examples do not constitute the majority of patients.

Similarly, the laboratory may play a critical role in establishing a diagnosis of sarcoidosis, syphilis, lymphoma, or toxoplasmosis, but the role of the lab should be confirmatory. Based on Bayes' Theorem,[1] one will be frequently misled by laboratory tests if they are applied in a screening fashion.

Dermatology is perhaps the one clinical subspecialty that relies more on the examination than the history. Most patients just do not have the vocabulary to convey as much information about a rash as a skilled practitioner gains with a glance at the pathology. Ophthalmology approaches dermatology with the ability to "see" the problem, but even the most skilled ophthalmologist cannot see suddenness of onset, duration, continuity, or systemic symptoms.

Give us one tool, and we will take the history hands down over our slit lamp, our indirect, and our lab. Maybe we need to do the study and compare 2 ophthalmologists for diagnostic accuracy, allowing one the chance to chat and the other the chance to look. Our guess is that the ears and tongue will outperform the eyes.

Reference

1. Rosenbaum JT, Wernick R. The utility of routine screening of patients with uveitis for systemic lupus erythematosus or tuberculosis. A Bayesian analysis. *Arch Ophthalmol.* 1990;108:1291-1293.

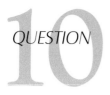

QUESTION

WHAT IS THE RISK OF BLINDNESS DUE TO UVEITIS IN PATIENTS TREATED WITH STEROID MONOTHERAPY?

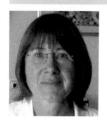

Aniki Rothova, MD, PhD

Before answering this question, let me evaluate its separate parts:

- What is the general risk of blindness in uveitis?
- What is the effect of the various treatment modalities on visual acuity?
- What are the side effects of the various treatments used?
- What is the specific effect of corticosteroids on uveitis and vision?

What Is the General Risk of Blindness in Uveitis?

Noninfectious uveitis is a major contributor to blindness and is a visual handicap in the working population (6% to 15%; depending on the geographical area). The chance of developing a blind eye depends on the anatomical type of uveitis, specific diagnoses, and development of complications either as a consequence of the disease itself or its treatment. The risk rate of developing a blind eye due to noninfectious uveitis has not yet been systematically studied in a large series and depends on its specific cause. The syndromes associated with poor visual prognosis include birdshot chorioretinopathy, Behçet's disease, and juvenile idiopathic arthritis (although a better prognosis was noted, for example, for human leukocyte antigen [HLA] B27-associated uveitis, and Fuchs' heterochromic uveitis syndrome). The exact risk of developing blindness in specific uveitis disorders is not known. The prevalence of at least one legally blind eye (vision less than 0.1) in a trans-sectional uveitis series from tertiary centers was 13% to 14%, and the prevalence of bilateral blindness was approximately 4%.[1,2] However, patients with uveitis typically suffer from prolonged periods of inflammatory activity associated with low vision, although their optimal visual acuity might remain uncompromised.[3] In this way, uveitis is a major cause of disability and compromised quality of life in relatively young patients. Prolonged visual loss occurred in two-thirds of uveitis patients, and 22% of patients met the criteria for legal blindness at some point in their follow-up. The most frequent causes of visual loss in uveitis include cystoid macular edema and cataract.[1-3]

What Is the Effect of the Various Treatment Modalities on Visual Acuity?

The patients with noninfectious uveitis are usually primarily treated using a step ladder approach with topical and periocular treatment modalities first and with systemic treatment regimens with immunomodulating drugs including corticosteroids, cytostatics, and biologics in severe and/or nonresponding cases.[4] Current response rates appear much better than in earlier trials, presumably because of recently developed, novel, nonsteroid therapies. The association between the specific treatment modalities and visual prognosis is not known. In contrast to other regimens, there are no data on sustained remissions of chronic uveitis achieved by systemic use of steroids solely.

What Are the Side Effects of the Various Treatments Used?

The frequency and severity of side effects during short periods (several weeks) of corticosteroid administration are limited, in contrast to its long-term use, which is associated with multiple systemic effects also observed among adults taking low-to-medium doses. Long-term use of systemic steroids is characterized by widely known adverse effects, including growth retardation, obesity, diabetes mellitus, osteopenia, and many others. A study comparing the adverse effects of steroids to immunosuppressive drugs in patients with ocular disorders revealed that the adverse effects and subsequent morbidity were more severe in the corticosteroid-treated group.[5] In the Systemic Immunosuppressive Therapy for Eye Diseases Cohort (SITE) study, 2340 patients with uveitis were treated with immunosuppressive drugs. The study has revealed that the most commonly used immunosuppressive drugs do not seem to increase overall mortality or mortality due to cancer; the alkylating agents and tumor necrosis factor alpha inhibitors might have increased overall mortality, but definitive conclusions were precluded by the limited number of patients who were treated with these drugs.[6]

What Is the Specific Effect of Corticosteroids on Uveitis and Vision?

Corticosteroids are characterized by their quick effect on the activity of inflammation, and their timely administration might be the quickest way to achieve a well-controlled uveitis. While systemic steroids quickly reduce active intraocular inflammatory signs, no systematic data are available on their long-term efficacy and visual acuity.[7] If the ocular inflammation is chronic or recurrent, systemic steroids are not recommended primarily because of the high frequency of corticosteroid-induced side effects.[8] Data obtained from small studies on birdshot chorioretinopathy and Behçet's disease indicate that systemic steroids had no effect on the final visual prognosis in chronic uveitis entities.[9-11]

Personal View

I believe that while systemic steroids have a quick effect on inflammatory signs, they do not alter the long-term visual prognosis. To our residents, I would say that using the monotherapy with corticosteroids in chronic and severe uveitis means that the patients will probably go blind more comfortably. The main indication for steroids is as the quickest way to bring down the active signs of inflammation before the other medication can take over.

Summary

When uveitis attacks are infrequent, transitory, and mild, the occasional administration of systemic steroids is an acceptable approach. However, when attacks are more frequent or severe, the importance changes from lessening the symptoms to prevention of activity.

Corticosteroids are valuable for their quick effect and are indicated as an initial or short-term treatment, but are not suitable for long-term administration.

References

1. Rothova A, Suttorp-van Schulten MS, Frits Treffers W, Kijlstra A. Causes and frequency of blindness in patients with intraocular inflammatory disease. *Br J Ophthalmol.* 1996;80:332-336.
2. Khairallah M, Yahia SB, Ladjimi A, et al. Pattern of uveitis in a referral centre in Tunisia, North Africa. *Eye (London).* 2007;21:33-39. Epub 2006 Feb 17.
3. Durrani OM, Tehrani NN, Marr JE, Moradi P, Stavrou P, Murray PI. Degree, duration, and causes of visual loss in uveitis. *Br J Ophthalmol.* 2004;88:1159-1162.
4. Lee FF, Foster CS. Pharmacotherapy of uveitis. *Expert Opin Pharmacother.* 2010;11:1135-1146.
5. Tamesis RR, Rodriguez A, Christen WG, Akova YA, Messmer E, Foster CS. Systemic drug toxicity trends in immunosuppressive therapy of immune and inflammatory ocular disease. *Ophthalmology.* 1996;103:768-775.
6. Kempen JH, Daniel E, Dunn JP, et al. Overall and cancer related mortality among patients with ocular inflammation treated with immunosuppressive drugs: retrospective cohort study. *BMJ.* 2009;339:b2480.
7. Rothova A. Corticosteroids in uveitis. *Ophthalmol Clin North Am.* 2002;15:389-394.
8. Nguyen QD, Hatef E, Kayen B, et al. A cross-sectional study of the current treatment patterns in noninfectious uveitis among specialists in the United States. *Ophthalmology.* 2011;118:184-190.
9. Mamo JG. The rate of visual loss in Behçet's disease. *Arch Ophthalmol.* 1970;84:451-452.
10. Rothova A, Berendschot TT, Probst K, van Kooij B, Baarsma GS. Birdshot chorioretinopathy: long-term manifestations and visual prognosis. *Ophthalmology.* 2004;111:954-959.
11. Thorne JE, Jabs DA, Peters GB, Hair D, Dunn JP, Kempen JH. Birdshot retinochoroidopathy: ocular complications and visual impairment. *Am J Ophthalmol.* 2005;140:45-51.

HOW SHOULD ONE PROPERLY EMPLOY TOPICAL CORTICOSTEROID THERAPY?

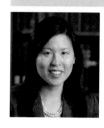

Olivia L. Lee, MD
(co-authored with C. Michael Samson, MD, MBA)

Corticosteroids have been in use for the treatment of noninfectious uveitis since the 1950s. Even today, corticosteroids remain the only Food and Drug Administration-approved medication for uveitis. Steroids can be administered topically, locally by injection or surgical intervention, orally, or intravenously. As ophthalmologists, we are all familiar and comfortable with the use of topical steroids to suppress ocular inflammation, such as in the postoperative setting. Therefore, it is not surprising that topical steroids are the mainstay and often the only form of immunosuppression that most ophthalmologists employ for the treatment of noninfectious uveitis.

Glucocorticoids have both anti-inflammatory and immunosuppressive properties, irrespective of the etiology of the inflammatory response (eg, traumatic, infectious, auto-immune, postsurgical, etc). By binding to intracellular steroid receptors, the medication inhibits production of phospholipase A2, thereby decreasing availability of arachidonic acid. The mechanism of action is thereby to inhibit production of potent mediators of inflammation: prostaglandins, thromboxanes, and leukotrienes. At a tissue level, gluco-corticoids prevent macrophage migration, reduce capillary permeability, suppress fibro-blast proliferation, and decrease vascular congestion. When systemically administered, the drug alters migration activity of T-cells and neutrophils. This phenomenon accounts for the decrease in inflammatory cells at the site of inflammation. These changes to the immune system are temporary and cease within days of discontinuing steroid use.

Various topical steroids are available for ophthalmic use; those that are currently available in the United States are listed in Table 11-1. Preparations with phosphate are hydro-philic and poorly penetrate intact corneal epithelium. Those steroids that contain alcohol or acetate are biphasic and penetrate intact cornea, the latter being the more potent. We prefer prednisolone acetate 1% (Pred Forte) for topical use in uveitis. The smaller

Table 11-1
Currently Available Topical Corticosteroid Ophthalmic Medications*

Steroid	Trade Name
Difluprednate 0.05%	Durezol
Prednisolone acetate 1%	Generic, Pred Forte, Omnipred
Dexamethasone 0.1%	Generic
Fluorometholone 0.25%	FML Forte
Fluorometholone 0.1%	Generic, FML, Flarex
Rimexolone 1%	Vexol
Medrysone 1%	HMS
Prednisolone acetate 0.125%	Pred Mild
Loteprednol 0.5%	Lotemax
Loteprednol 0.2%	Alrex

*Listed in order of highest (top) to lowest (bottom) potency.

particle size and slower sedimentation may explain better bioavailability[1], accounting for improved therapeutic response seen in some patients when switching from generic. Not uncommonly, our patients are instructed to apply this medication every 1 to 2 hours while awake during an acute episode of severe anterior uveitis. The patient should be reminded to shake the bottle prior to use. Difluprednate 0.05% (Durezol) is a newly available topical steroid with which 4 times daily dosing with is equivalent to Pred Forte 8 times daily.[2] This is particularly useful and convenient for patients who have difficulty complying with hourly dosing schedules.

When prescribing topical steroids, it is important to be cognizant of potential side effects, both common and rare. Ocular effects such as increased intraocular pressure (IOP) and cataract formation are well recognized by ophthalmologists. Topical steroids can also cause ptosis, mydriasis, sclera melt, and eyelid skin atrophy. Steroid-induced IOP rise is variable amongst patients and high levels of IOP elevation are usually reproducible, even with modest steroid usage. Steroid responsiveness is seen 2 to 6 weeks after initiation of topical steroid use and can affect up to 25% of patients. However, infants and children can develop steroid responsiveness with rapid onset, often within 1.5 weeks of initiating steroid use. IOP-elevating potential varies between different steroid formulations, with difluprednate, dexamethasone, and prednisolone being associated with the highest rise in IOP. Steroids with less IOP-elevating potential include fluorometholone, rimexolone, and loteprednol. It is not advisable to lighten or discontinue steroid use in the face of IOP elevation when ocular inflammation remains uncontrolled. In this situation, glaucoma medication should be used to control IOP, and other means of inflammation control should be considered (ie, systemic steroids).

Although rare, systemic adverse effects can also be seen with isolated topical steroid use. Consequently, it is important for the ophthalmologist to recognize that steroids can cause hyperglycemia, hypertension, redistribution of fat (eg, moon faces, buffalo hump, central obesity), decreased bone density, aseptic necrosis of the hip, psychiatric changes (eg, psychosis), and peptic ulcer. One should be mindful of these effects in those patients with particular sensitivity, such as the elderly, diabetics, and infants or small children. A high systemic level of steroids during pregnancy leads to suppression of the hypothalamic-pituitary-adrenal axis and adrenal insufficiency in newborns. Systemic steroid use during pregnancy has also been associated with orofacial clefts.[3] Fortunately, topical steroids for ophthalmic use have not been reported in association with teratogenicity. We prefer to treat pregnant women with active uveitis with regional steroids, our preference being triamcinolone acetate (Kenalog or Triessence) administered by periocular or intravitreal injection. Another option for local therapy is Ozurdex, a sustained-release dexamethasone implant administered by intravitreal injection, which was approved for use in the treatment of noninfectious uveitis in 2010.

The choice of steroid formulation and dosing schedule should be tailored to the individual clinical scenario. Topical steroids are an excellent mode of treatment for certain uveitic conditions, especially as a first-line therapy for new-onset uveitis. For severe anterior chamber reaction, empirical aggressive topical steroid use is warranted if the diagnosis of noninfectious anterior uveitis is made. A typical regimen would include prednisolone acetate 1% every hour while awake, fluorometholone 0.1% ophthalmic ointment while asleep, along with a cycloplegic agent. In a patient with a proven history of autoimmune uveitis, a severe flare of anterior uveitis may be treated instead with periocular or systemic steroid and minimal concomitant topical steroid use. Once an improvement in cell and flare is observed, slow tapering of the steroid medication can begin. The patient should be monitored closely while tapering steroids, as reactivation may preclude tapering below a certain dose. A few drops a day may be tolerable for several weeks or more, particularly if the patient is not phakic nor a steroid responder. However, we prefer to consider immunosuppression for patients who continue to have recurrent episodes of uveitis or who are unable to be weaned off topical steroids.

In some situations, the use of topical steroids is not recommended. Reactivation of corneal herpetic disease is associated with topical steroid use and should be avoided if possible. Due to the risk of cataract formation associated with chronic topical steroid use, it is preferable to avoid 3 times daily or higher dosing of topical steroids in pediatric patients.[4] Therefore, in children with chronic anterior inflammation, such as juvenile idiopathic arthritis-associated uveitis, systemic treatment is usually necessary. In a patient with scleral or corneal thinning, topical steroids should be avoided as they may potentiate melting.

Topical steroids alone are insufficient treatment for autoimmune intermediate, posterior or panuveitis. First and foremost, infectious and malignant etiology should be considered, if not ruled out. Oral prednisone can be initiated at a dose of 1 to 1.5 mg/kg/day. While prolonged high dose systemic steroid use should be avoided, a reasonable duration of 1 or 2 weeks should be allowed to observe clinical improvement. Then a taper can be initiated. If the patient experiences intolerable adverse effects or is unable to taper below 10 mg of prednisone daily, systemic immunosuppression should be considered.[5] For long-term local steroid treatment, Retisert, an surgically implanted intravitreal implant, delivers fluocinolone for approximately 3 years. Retisert has been shown to have equivalent efficacy when compared to systemic therapy for the treatment of noninfectious intermediate, posterior and panuveitis.[6]

References

1. Roberts CW, Nelson PL. Comparative analysis of prednisolone acetate suspensions. *J Ocul Pharmacol Ther.* 2007;23:182-187.
2. Foster CS, Davanzo R, Flynn TE, McLeod K, Vogel R, Crockett RS. Durezol (difluprednate ophthalmic emulsion 0.05%) compared with Pred Forte 1% ophthalmic suspension in the treatment of endogenous anterior uveitis. *J Ocul Pharmacol Ther.* 2010;26:475-483.
3. Park-Wyllie L, Mazzotta P, Pastuszak A, et al. Birth defects after maternal exposure to corticosteroids: prospective cohort study and meta-analysis of epidemiological studies. *Teratology.* 2000;62:385-392.
4. Thorne JE, Woreta FA, Dunn JP, Jabs DA. Risk of cataract development among children with juvenile idiopathic arthritis-related uveitis treated with topical corticosteroids. *Ophthalmology.* 2010;117:1436-1441.
5. Jabs DA, Rosenbaum JT, Foster CS, et al. Guidelines for the use of immunosuppressive drugs in patients with ocular inflammatory disorders: recommendations of an expert panel. *Am J Ophthalmol.* 2000;130:492-513.
6. Kempen JH, Altaweel MM, Holbrook JT, et al; Multicenter Uveitis Steroid Treatment (MUST) Trial Research Group. Randomized comparison of systemic anti-inflammatory therapy versus fluocinolone acetonide implant for intermediate, posterior, and panuveitis: the multicenter uveitis steroid treatment trial. *Ophthalmology.* 2011;118:1916-1926.

IS THERE A DIFFERENCE BETWEEN THE VARIOUS TOPICAL CORTICOSTEROID PREPARATIONS?

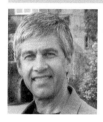

Joseph Tauber, MD

Recommendations for intelligent prescribing of topical corticosteroids must first be placed in context. There are certain clinical scenarios in which no topical corticosteroid preparation is likely to be effective. Limited intraocular penetration and bioavailability explains why, even when applied very frequently, topical corticosteroids will be inadequate to control intermediate or posterior inflammatory conditions. Regional injections or systemic treatment are more appropriate and effective routes for corticosteroid therapy of such disorders. Topical preparations of corticosteroids can be dramatically effective in treatment of mild to marked degrees of inflammation affecting the conjunctiva and/or anterior segment. In my experience, there are clear differences between available topical preparations of corticosteroids, and clinicians can maximize the likelihood of prompt control of inflammation with a minimum of side effects by learning the nuances of their use. Clinicians must learn to balance potency of anti-inflammatory efficacy, comfort, cost, and side effect profile of each formulation.

Because corticosteroids in various formulations are used to treat diverse human diseases, scales have been prepared ranking the potency of corticosteroid molecules, particularly for dermatologic disease. Unfortunately, these scales are of little guidance in treating inflammatory disease of the eye. With respect to ocular disease, potency depends on local bioavailability, which depends on solubility, intra-bottle clumping, ocular surface retention time, and speed of metabolic breakdown. Numerous studies of endogenous and postoperative inflammation have led to the widely held view that, with respect to potency of anti-inflammatory activity, prednisolone acetate is the gold standard of topical preparations. Disadvantages of this molecule (in the short term) include its suspension formulation and the risk of ocular hypertension. Discussion of the side effects of chronic corticosteroid use is beyond the scope of this chapter. Despite several published studies in postcataract surgery models of inflammation showing comparable efficacy between prednisolone (Pred Forte or Econopred Plus) and other generic preparations,[1,2] my personal experience, and that of many other ocular immunology specialists, is that the brand name formulation Pred Forte offers significantly better anti-inflammatory efficacy than any other pred-nisolone acetate preparation. This is most evident in patients with uveitis who suffer higher levels of inflammation than are typically seen following cataract surgery. Some have speculated that the apparent inferiority of generic preparations is due to greater clumping of dry particles within the bottle in generic preparations, leading to reduced delivered drug concentration per drop.[1,3,4] Despite repeated claims by manufacturers that a "new and improved milling process" has solved the clumping issue, my experience has been that notably more clumping, reduced patient comfort, and superficial keratitis occurs with generic formulations. I believe Pred Forte retains a justified place as the gold standard of topical corticosteroid preparations. Mention must be made of the efficacy of topical loteprednol (LE) in patients at higher risk for elevated intraocular pressure (IOP). While no head-to-head comparison is available, many clinicians feel that LE is nearly as potent as Pred Forte and has a much lower incidence of elevated intraocular pressure. Earlier topical preparations of rimexolone and fluorometholone offered a reduced incidence of IOP complications, but with markedly reduced anti-inflammatory efficacy. LE is a reasonable option as a first-choice corticosteroid for all but severe inflammatory disorders and should be the first replacement for prednisolone acetate in patients with significant steroid-induced elevation of intraocular pressure. Disadvantages of LE include slightly suboptimal anti-inflammatory efficacy and the lack of a generic alternative. I have had many patients with corneal graft rejection episodes that were uncontrolled with LE, which responded when therapy was switched to prednisolone acetate. In my practice, when drug cost is a significant barrier for patients, fluorometholone may be substituted instead. Fluorinated corticosteroid preparations hold the potential for greater anti-inflammatory efficacy, consistent with what is observed in systemic use.[5]

Difluprednate is the most recently approved topical ocular corticosteroid formulation and incorporates 2 fluorine molecules. Studies in uveitis and postcataract surgery inflammation showed equivalent anti-inflammatory efficacy to Pred Forte even with less frequent difluprednate dosing (twice daily versus 4 times daily). Few large studies have been published other than those included in the Food and Drug Administration submission.[6] Nonetheless, I have found difluprednate to be excellent with respect to clinical efficacy, and I have been successful in bringing high levels of intraocular inflammation under control. Potential disadvantages of difluprednate include reports of ocular hypertension, variable patient tolerance, and cost. One report described ocular hypertension occurring more rapidly in difluprednate-treated patients than has been described following prednisolone acetate therapy.[7] Further study is needed to reliably rank topical corticosteroid preparations in a meaningful way regarding efficacy and risk of serious side effects.

References

1. Gayton JL. A clinical comparison of two different prednisolone acetate formulations in patients undergoing cataract surgery. *Curr Med Res Opin.* 2005;21:1291-1295.
2. Samudre SS, Lattanzio FA Jr, Williams PB, Sheppard JD Jr. Comparison of topical steroids for acute anterior uveitis. *J Ocul Pharmacol Ther.* 2004;20:533-547.
3. Roberts CW, Nelson PL. Comparative analysis of prednisolone acetate suspensions. *J Ocul Pharmacol Ther.* 2007;23:182-187.
4. Fiscella RG, Jensen M, Van Dyck G. Generic prednisolone suspension substitution. *Arch Ophthalmol.* 1998;116:703.
5. Bikowski J, Pillai R, Shroot B. The position not the presence of the halogen in corticosteroids influences potency and side effects. *J Drugs Dermatol.* 2006;5:125-130.
6. Korenfeld MS, Silverstein SM, Cooke DL, et al. Difluprednate ophthalmic emulsion 0.05% for postoperative inflammation and pain. *J Cataract Refract Surg.* 2009;35:26-34.
7. Cable M. Intraocular pressure spikes using difluprednate 0.05% for postoperative cataract inflammation. Program 1981. Paper presented at: Association for Research in Vision and Ophthalmology Annual Meeting; May 30, 2010; Fort Lauderdale, FL.

How Do I Establish a Diagnosis When I Suspect Sarcoidosis to Be the Cause of Uveitis?

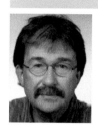

Manfred Zierhut, MD, PhD

Approximately 30% to 60% of patients with sarcoidosis develop ophthalmic manifestations. Bilateral granulomatous uveitis is the most frequent presentation. If sarcoidosis is suspected as the cause of uveitis, the final goal has to be a confirming biopsy leading to "definite sarcoidosis with ocular involvement." The biopsy discloses noncaseating granulomatous inflammation. However, a biopsy is often impossible to perform because no location of pathology is detectable. Therefore, various degrees of certainty have recently led to *International Criteria for the Diagnosis of Ocular Sarcoidosis.*[1]

It seems that most of the patients with sarcoidosis uveitis have no severe lung or other organ involvement. Therefore, the history should exclude dyspnea, fever attacks, and night sweats.

The most important suspicion of sarcoidosis uveitis comes from the clinical findings (Table 13-1). The *International Criteria* summarize these findings.

The association of snow balls and peripheral chorioretinal lesions and anterior synechiae (Figure 13-1) in my opinion are very suggestive of sarcoid uveitis (with a very limited differential diagnosis of tuberculosis [TB]), as are iris nodules (Figure 13-2), macroaneurysms, and optic disc granuloma (Figure 13-3).

After the clinical investigation, you should continue with laboratory investigations, and Table 13-2 shows the suggested ones.

It is unclear at this moment what type of TB test should be done to exclude TB. I suggest using the Quantiferon-test, which would be negative in case of Bacillus Calmette-Guérin (BCG) vaccination. In case we have a high suspicion for sarcoid because of clinical findings, we go on directly to the more sensitive computed tomography (CT) scan, without

Table 13-1
Clinical Signs Suggestive of Ocular Sarcoidosis

1. Mutton fat keratic precipitates and/or iris nodules at pupillary margin or on stroma.
2. Trabecular meshwork nodules and/or tent-shaped peripheral anterior synechiae.
3. Snowballs/strings of pearls of vitreous opacities.
4. Multifocal peripheral chorioretinal lesions (active and atrophic).
5. Nodular and/or segmental periphlebitis (with or without candle wax exudate) and/or macroaneurysm.
6. Optic disc nodules/granuloma and/or solitary choroidal nodule.
7. Bilateral inflammation.

Adapted from Herbort CP, Mochizuki M, Rao NA; Scientific Committee of the First International Workshop on Ocular Sarcoidosis (IWOS). International criteria for the diagnosis of ocular sarcoidosis: results of the first international workshop on ocular sarcoidosis (IWOS). *Ocul Immunol Inflamm.* 2009;17:160-169.

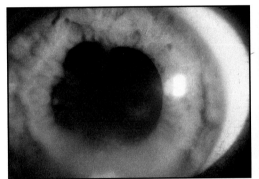

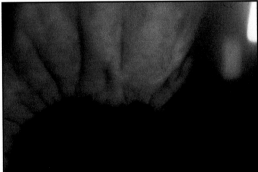

Figure 13-1. Anterior synechiae from 2 to 5 o'clock.

Figure 13-2. Iris with pupillary nodules.

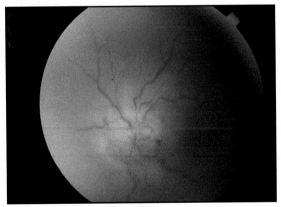

Figure 13-3. Optic disc edema.

Table 13-2
Laboratory Investigations in Suspected Ocular Sarcoidosis

1. Negative tuberculin test
2. Elevated serum angiotensin-converting enzyme and/or elevated serum lysozyme
3. Chest x-ray: bilateral hilar lymphadenopathy
4. Abnormal liver enzyme tests (any 2 of: alkaline phosphatase, aspartate transaminases, alanine transaminases)
5. Chest CT scan in patients with normal chest x-ray

Adapted from Herbort CP, Mochizuki M, Rao NA; Scientific Committee of the First International Workshop on Ocular Sarcoidosis (IWOS). International criteria for the diagnosis of ocular sarcoidosis: results of the first international workshop on ocular sarcoidosis (IWOS). *Ocul Immunol Inflamm.* 2009;17:160-169.

Table 13-3
Diagnostic Criteria for Ocular Sarcoidosis

1. Biopsy-supported diagnosis with compatible uveitis	Definite ocular sarcoidosis
2. Biopsy not done, bilateral hilar lymphadenopathy with compatible uveitis	Presumed ocular sarcoidosis
3. Biopsy not done, chest x-ray normal; 3 suggestive ocular signs and 2 positive investigational tests	Probable ocular sarcoidosis
4. Biopsy negative; 4 suggestive ocular findings and 2 positive investigations	Possible ocular sarcoidosis

Adapted from Herbort CP, Mochizuki M, Rao NA; Scientific Committee of the First International Workshop on Ocular Sarcoidosis (IWOS). International criteria for the diagnosis of ocular sarcoidosis: results of the first international workshop on ocular sarcoidosis (IWOS). *Ocul Immunol Inflamm.* 2009;17:160-169.

x-ray. Bronchoalveolar lavage or transbronchial lung biopsy may then allow harvesting cells. Gallium scan is less often used, as a panel of experts has recently communicated.[2] It is replaced by positron emission tomography (PET)/CT scan at least in some countries. As a general rule, we try to use imaging methods only when the actual corticosteroid dosage is very low because the granulomas of a low-grade sarcoidosis would quickly disappear in chest x-ray and even CT scan under this treatment. This is the case before any anti-inflammatory treatment starts or before the dosage is increased due to recurrence.

The combination of clinical and laboratory findings then allows you to name your diagnosis adequately (Table 13-3).

There are countries, like Japan, with a higher incidence of sarcoid uveitis, making it more likely to suspect sarcoidosis when the clinical signs and the laboratory findings are not conclusive, leading at least to the category of "possible ocular sarcoidosis." You also should be aware that general sarcoidosis may develop in the following years. Therefore, you have to keep in mind that repetition of the laboratory tests periodically is appropriate.

The determination of a soluble interleukin (IL)-2 receptor is playing an increasing role in the diagnosis of sarcoidosis, being more specific than the angiotensin-converting enzyme (ACE). In a revised version of the previously mentioned criteria, this parameter may replace ACE in the future.

The diagnosis of sarcoidosis in young patients is even more difficult. In this age, the presenting sign often is arthritis. With increasing age, the likelihood of lung involvement increases. Angiotensin-converting enzyme also is typically elevated in children, so this is not really helpful as a diagnostic marker. Sarcoid-induced uveitis in childhood may mimic the uveitis of juvenile idiopathic arthritis.

I personally also think of sarcoidosis when I see a very quick response to systemic corticosteroids (prednisolone 1 mg/kg for 1 week, reduction for 10 mg per week). In case where I cannot identify any associated disease, but cannot prove sarcoid, I would use this idea as a working hypothesis but would have to be aware of any other new findings, like multiple sclerosis in case of intermediate uveitis.

References

1. Herbort CP, Mochizuki M, Rao NA; Scientific Committee of the First International Workshop on Ocular Sarcoidosis (IWOS). International criteria for the diagnosis of ocular sarcoidosis: results of the first international workshop on ocular sarcoidosis. *Ocul Immunol Inflamm.* 2009;17:160-169.
2. Wakefield D, Zierhut M. Controversy: ocular sarcoidosis. *Ocul Immunol Inflamm.* 2010;18:5-9.

When and How Should Intermediate Uveitis Be Treated?

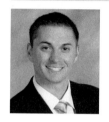

John Randolph, MD
(co-authored with Henry J. Kaplan, MD)

Intermediate uveitis refers to inflammation in the vitreous cavity, commonly with involvement of the peripheral retina and/or pars plana.[1] The decision of when and how to treat intermediate uveitis is guided by several principles that, when properly applied, control inflammation and preserve vision in the overwhelming majority of eyes.

The first goal in treating intermediate uveitis is to identify the underlying etiology. The etiology of intermediate uveitis falls into 1 of 4 categories: 1) idiopathic or pars planitis, 2) infectious (eg, tuberculosis, syphilis, Lyme disease), 3) autoimmune (eg, multiple sclerosis, sarcoidosis, Behçet's disease), and 4) neoplastic (eg, non-Hodgkin's lymphoma). Only after arriving at a correct diagnosis should a targeted approach to treatment be initiated. For example, infections such as syphilis and tuberculosis are treated with appropriate antimicrobial medications, whereas anti-inflammatory agents are preferred for autoimmune entities such as sarcoidosis and Behçet's disease.

Selected diagnostic tests are only performed when: 1) suggested by the history and/or clinical presentation (eg, Lyme disease), or 2) when medical and/or surgical treatment will be altered by the diagnosis (eg, diagnostic pars plana vitrectomy for non-Hodgkin's lymphoma).

Treatment of pars planitis (ie, idiopathic intermediate uveitis) should be guided by the visual demands of the patient or the development of ocular complications. Although a visual acuity of 20/40 or worse was the classic indication to initiate treatment, it is probably inappropriate today. For example, a patient with 20/20 visual acuity with floaters that interfere with function or that are symptomatically disabling should be treated; in contrast, an asymptomatic patient with 20/40 acuity need not necessarily be treated. Complications that should result in the initiation of treatment are newly established cystoid macular edema, symptomatic vitreo-macular traction (Figure 14-1), posterior

Figure 14-1. Optical coherence tomography demonstrating vitreo-macular traction with associated macular edema.

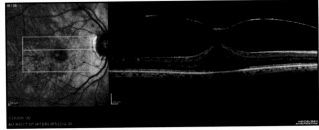

Figure 14-2. Fundus photograph demonstrating inferior pars plana snowbanking.

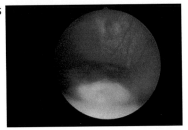

subcapsular cataract, inferior retinoschisis, and peripheral neovascularization causing vitreous hemorrhage.

As a general principle, we recommend a 4-step approach for the treatment of idiopathic intermediate uveitis[2]:

- *Step 1:* Corticosteroids: Treatment may be administered in the form of either systemic or injectable (periocular or intravitreal) corticosteroids. The age of the patient should be considered when deciding the route of administration. Although the side effect profile of systemic corticosteroids is better tolerated in younger patients, the potential for retardation of growth requires very careful monitoring.

  For those patients presenting with monocular inflammation, we prefer periocular or intravitreal triamcinolone acetonide injections (40 mg in 1 cc or 4 mg in 0.1 cc, respectively) at 6-week intervals until inflammation is controlled.

  In the setting of binocular inflammation, we most frequently start systemic corticosteroid therapy. Oral corticosteroids are administered at a dose of 1 mg/kg/day in 4 divided doses for 2 weeks. If the patient responds within 4 weeks, a gradual taper of 10 to 20 mg per week is employed with the goal of controlling inflammation at a dose of 10 mg a day or less. Intravitreal or periocular triamcinolone acetonide may be used in conjunction with oral steroids as described previously.

- *Step 2:* If corticosteroid therapy fails to control inflammation, ablative therapy with cryotherapy or laser photocoagulation is preferred.

  Cryotherapy is performed by first creating an inferior 180 degree conjunctival peritomy and isolating the inferior rectus and horizontal rectus muscles, thus allowing unabated access to the inferior retina/snowbank (Figure 14-2). Three rows of cryopexy are applied using a freeze-thaw technique with timing of ice ball formation on the retina without a snowbank. Treatment of the snowbank area is then timed, because it is not possible to visualize the ice ball in a snowbank. Treatment extends for the full extent of the snowbank and involves placing 3 separate rows of cryotherapy—one anterior to the snowbank, a second overlying the snowbank, and a third row just posterior to the snowbank. The main advantage of cryotherapy lies in the ability to directly treat the pars plana snowbank. Following cryotherapy, approximately 50% of patients will demonstrate complete remission, with the remainder entering a quiescent phase lasting 1 to 3 years.

Peripheral laser photocoagulation may also be used by placing 3 to 4 confluent rows of burns just posterior to the snowbank. Treatment is extended 1 clock hour superior to the snowbank on either side.[3] Efficacy appears to be comparable to cryotherapy; however, direct treatment to the pars plana snowbank is not possible with this technique.

- *Step 3:* Should ablative therapy fail, small-gauge pars plana vitrectomy (23 or 25 ga) with separation and removal of the posterior hyaloid and peripheral laser photocoagulation is our treatment of choice. Vitrectomy is also indicated in cases of visual loss due to dense vitreous debris, chronic vitreous hemorrhage, medically nonresponsive cystoid macular edema, and relief of peripheral retinal traction associated with inferior retinoschisis.

- *Step 4:* If inflammation continues or recurs, we then prescribe systemic immunomodulatory therapy (IMT). We generally start with oral methotrexate used in combination with a systemic corticosteroid taper as outlined in Step 1. Additional agents to consider include purine antagonists (eg, azathioprine), cytotoxic drugs (eg, cyclophosphamide), calcineurin modulators (eg, cyclosporine), or anti-TNF agents (eg, infliximab, etanercept, or adalimumab). Anecdotal clinical reports suggest that new biologic agents, such as anti-tumor necrosis factor drugs, may be effective and comparatively well-tolerated options in the treatment of refractory uveitis in the short term. However, the uncertainty of their long-term results coupled with their high cost and need for repeated parenteral use have limited their widespread adoption.[4]

References

1. Lai WW, Pulido JS. Intermediate uveitis. *Ophthalmol Clin North Am.* 2002;15:309-317.
2. Kaplan HJ. Intermediate uveitis (pars planitis, chronic cyclitis)—a four step approach to treatment. In: Saari KM, ed. *Uveitis Update.* Amsterdam, Netherlands: Excerpta Medica; 1984:169-172.
3. Park SE, Mieler WF, Pulido JS. Peripheral scatter photocoagulation for neovascularization associated with pars planitis. *Arch Ophthalmol.* 1995;113:1277-1280.
4. Jap A, Chee SP. Immunosuppressive therapy for ocular diseases. *Curr Opin Ophthalmol.* 2008;19:535-540.

WHAT ARE SOME IMPORTANT ASSOCIATIONS BETWEEN HUMAN LEUKOCYTE ANTIGEN PHENOTYPES AND SPECIFIC UVEITIS SYNDROMES?

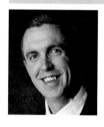

Mark S. Dacey, MD

Human leukocyte antigens (HLA) are inherited antigens that are present on the surface of nucleated cells within the human body. HLA represents the major histocompatibility complex (MHC) and is encoded for by genes on chromosome 6. MHC is involved in several crucial functions, including antigen presentation, prediction of graft rejection, and autoimmunity. There are a number of clinical associations between various HLA phenotypes and ocular inflammatory conditions that influence diagnosis and treatment strategies.[1]

HLA antigens may correspond to MHC class I or II. MHC Class I (A, B, and C) involves presentation of fragments of intracellular proteins to the cellular surface, which subsequently attract CD-8+ T-cells. Conversely, MHC class II (DP, DQ, and DR) present peptides from antigens outside of the cell, which attract helper T-cells.

Clinical evaluation of HLA typing, including both class I and II (A, B, C, DP, DQ, DR), is an essential tool in assessing the differential diagnosis in patients with ocular inflammation. Within the differential diagnosis, I order HLA typing on my patients in an effort to not only diagnose their ocular condition, but to provide information regarding familial risk.

HLA is essential in the evaluation of noninfectious posterior uveitis and retinal vasculitis. The strongest association ever described between HLA and disease exists with the HLA-A29 phenotype and birdshot retinochoroidopathy (BSRC), conferring a relative risk of 50 to 224. Feltkamp[2] calculated that the diagnosis of BSRC rises from 70% to 97% in HLA-A29-positive patients and decreases from 70% to 8.5% in HLA-A29-negative patients. HLA-A29 has 2 separate alleles, A29.1 and A29.2, which differ by a single base pair substitution. The A29.2 allele is found in 90% of Northern European Whites, whereas

A29.1 is present most often in Southeast Asian patients. Only the A29.2 allele is present in BSRC patients, leading to the theory that A29.1 might impair the T-cell activation that is crucial in BSRC pathogenesis. However, the presence of HLA-A29 does not imply that the patient will develop BSRC; only 11% of HLA-A29-positive controls developed the disease. Additional HLA associations in posterior uveitis include HLA-B51 with Adamantiades-Behçet's disease and HLA-DR4 (specifically DRB1*0405) with Vogt-Koyanagi-Harada's disease.

HLA is also widely used in the evaluation of intermediate uveitis. HLA-DR2 and DR15 both confer a relative risk of approximately 3 in the development of pars planitis, while HLA-B8 and B51 have recently been identified as MHC class I risk factors. Multiple sclerosis (MS) is frequently associated with pars planitis. Similarly, DR2 and DR15 (specifically DRB1*1501) have also been associated with the development of MS in Northern European populations independent of the development of pars planitis. Recently, HLA-B7 has also been associated with the development of symptomatic uveitis in MS patients.

HLA-B27 is a critical tool in the evaluation of acute anterior nongranulomatous uveitis, with 40% to 60% of these patients estimated to be HLA-B27 positive. Conversely, only 1.4% to 8.0% of the general population carries this allele, conferring a relative risk of 15. In my experience, HLA-B27-positive uveitis patients have a disease course that is more resistant to therapy and have more frequent recurrences, with a higher percentage requiring immunomodulatory therapy to prevent episodes. A positive test for B27 should trigger the clinician to evaluate for the associated seronegative spondylarthropathies. Anterior uveitis develops in 25% to 30% of patients with ankylosing spondylitis, 20% to 30% with psoriatic arthritis, 25% with Reiter's syndrome, and 2% to 11% of patients with inflammatory bowel disease.[3] In a Japanese study, HLA-DR8 was found to be associated with acute anterior uveitis but not with ankylosing spondylitis.[4]

The risk of development and prognosis for chronic anterior uveitis in patients with juvenile idiopathic arthritis (JIA) is associated with several loci of MHC class II, specifically alleles HLA-DR5, DR11 (DRB1*1104, a split product of HLA-DR5), and DR13. HLA-DR8 has been associated with the development of JIA but has not been evaluated as an association of JIA-related uveitis.

Tubulointerstitial nephritis and uveitis (TINU) is a rare clinical entity representing a subset of patients with interstitial nephritis. The combination of HLA alleles DQ1, DQ5, and DR1 have been associated with the development of TINU, occurring in 72% of patients.

HLA typing is an extremely valuable test in assessing anterior, intermediate, and posterior uveitis. In particular, patients can be accurately diagnosed earlier in a given disease process through the use of HLA typing. For example, in evaluating a patient with retinal vasculitis, a strong suspicion for BSRC may be raised through a positive HLA-A29 test, and that patient may then be treated with immunomodulatory chemotherapy earlier in his or her clinical course. HLA testing enables clinicians to evaluate for associated systemic conditions before clinical manifestations occur, potentially allowing an opportunity to alter the disease course.

References

1. Krieglstein G, Weinreb R, Pleyer U, Foster CS. *Uveitis and Immunological Disorders*. Berlin, Germany: Springer-Verlag; 2007:103-106.
2. Feltkamp TE. HLA and uveitis. *Int Ophthalmol*. 1990;14:327-333.
3. Vitale A, Foster CS. *Diagnosis and Treatment of Uveitis*. Philadelphia, PA: WB Saunders Company; 2002.
4. Monowarul Islam SM, Numaga J, Fujino Y, et al. HLA-DR8 and acute anterior uveitis in ankylosing spondylitis. *Arthritis Rheum*. 1995;38:547-550.

How Do I Diagnose and Treat Herpetic Uveitis?

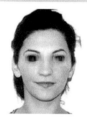

Dorine Makhoul, MD

Infections with viruses of the family *Herpesviridae* are common worldwide. More than 100 herpes viruses have been characterized, but only 8 infect humans: Herpes simplex virus (HSV) 1 and 2, varicella zoster virus (VZV), cytomegalovirus (CMV), Epstein–Barr virus (EBV), human herpes virus 6-7-8. Those viruses can cause a wide spectrum of ocular disease, which comprises a number of clinical presentations: blepharitis, keratoconjunctivitis, dendritic epithelial keratitis, geographic or trophic herpetic corneal ulceration, stromal keratitis, and intraocular inflammation. Intraocular herpetic inflammation can be divided into 2 major entities, anterior uveitis with or without active epithelial keratitis or interstitial keratitis and viral retinopathy, which were described in both immunocompetent and immunocompromised patients.

Anterior uveitis is the most common form of intraocular inflammation accounting for more than 90% of uveitis, and herpetic anterior uveitis either due to herpes simplex or varicella zoster virus infection accounts for 5% to 10% of all uveitis cases and is the most common cause of anterior infectious uveitis.

Diagnosis of Herpetic Anterior Uveitis

Because not all clinicians have access to intraocular fluid analysis, awareness of the clinical symptoms of herpetic anterior uveitis is important for diagnosis and subsequent

Figure 16-1. Inferior granulomatous keratic precipitates.

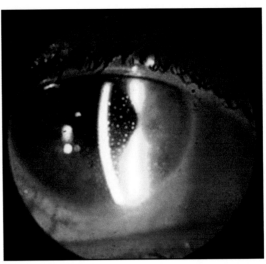

treatment. The diagnosis is relatively simple in the presence of concomitant skin lesions, active keratitis, and/or corneal anesthesia. However, in the absence of unclear evidence of current or past HSV infection, the diagnosis requires clinical suspicion and astute observations borne of such suspicion. Anterior uveitis secondary to HSV or VZV occurs in association with active or inactive corneal involvement, but anterior uveitis without associated corneal changes also occurs as an isolated entity.

Ocular involvement is virtually always unilateral, with patients suffering from blurry vision, photophobia, pain, and redness. On slit-lamp examination, we may find an active keratitis, corneal scaring, or normal cornea. The degree of intraocular inflammation can vary from mild to severe.

The iritis may be nongranulomatous but is more often granulomatous with moderate size mutton fat keratic precipitates (Figure 16-1), often in a triangular shape, located on the inferior part of the cornea, and, in the case of active keratitis, collects frequently under the area of the corneal lesion. Posterior synechiae, loss of the function of the sphincter muscles, and atrophy of the iris are responsible for a distorted pupil. The iris atrophy, which results from ischemic necrosis of the stroma, is characterized by a defect at the level of the iris pigment epithelium, has well-defined edges, and can be only seen with transillumination. It is in the specific search for such pathology via retroillumination that most ophthalmologists fail due to their lack of clinical suspicion for viral uveitis. Increased intraocular pressure is found in 90% of the patients, and trabeculitis is considered as the principal cause. Episcleritis and scleritis occur with anterior uveitis in less than 1% of patients.

The diagnosis of herpetic anterior uveitis is usually based on the previously mentioned clinical features, but the gold standard is the isolation of the virus or viral antigens in intraocular liquid as aqueous humor, which is obtained after an anterior chamber tap or vitreous fluid in case of posterior involvement. Serological testing for anti-HSV is a useful epidemiological tool but is not diagnostically helpful in an individual patient.

Confirmation of intraocular viral infection with or without viral replication relies on molecular techniques such as polymerase chain reaction (PCR). The sensitivity of PCR to detect viral DNA can reach 80% to 96%, and it requires a small quantity of intraocular fluid. A less widely used method for the diagnosis of herpetic uveitis is the Goldmann-Witmer (GW) coefficient. This coefficient compares the ratio of anti-herpes antibody in serum and aqueous humor with the ratio of total immunoglobulin G in serum and aqueous humor, and is considered positive if the ratio is greater than 3. The GW coefficient is more useful in immunocompetent patients because of the high false-negative rate in immunocompromised hosts.

Treatment of Herpetic Uveitis

The pathogenesis of herpetic iridocyclitis is believed to involve active viral replication and the host immune responses.

Topical corticosteroids and antiviral agents are commonly used to treat ocular herpetic disease. Topical corticosteroids control the iridocyclitis and also acutely decrease intraocular pressure owing to their anti-inflammatory effects on trabecular meshwork. However, topical and oral antihypertensive agents may be necessary to control the pressure especially initially.

Corticosteroids should be slowly tapered once the inflammation is controlled to avoid "the rebound effect." Topical antiviral agents promote resolution of herpetic epithelial keratitis, but their effect in deeper forms of ocular involvement has not been established. They should be used in concomitance with corticosteroid drops to prevent recurrent epithelial keratitis. The topical anti-herpetic agent of choice has become gancyclovir gel.

Concerning the use of oral acyclovir, the HEDS (herpetic eye disease control group) results suggest a benefit of oral acyclovir in the treatment of herpetic iridocyclitis in patients receiving topical corticosteroids and topical antiviral prophylaxis. Oral acyclovir at a dosage of 400 mg 5 times per day for several weeks is usually used. Intravenous acyclovir (10 mg/kg/d) may be considered in severe anterior uveitis and must be employed in all immunocompromised patients. Alternatively, one may use valacyclovir 1 g 3 times per day or famciclovir 500 mg 3 times daily. Oral acyclovir, 600 to 800 mg/day, given on a long-term basis, can diminish the recurrence of herpetic anterior uveitis.

I am not going to detail the viral retinopathies that are covered elsewhere in this work, but one must, for every anterior viral uveitis case, perform a dilated eye fundus to exclude any posterior involvement as an acute retinal necrosis or a progressive outer retinal necrosis syndrome.

Suggested Readings

Siverio Júnior CD, Imai Y, Cunningham ET Jr. Diagnosis and management of herpetic anterior uveitis. *Int Ophthalmol Clin.* 2002;42:43-48.

Sungur GK, Hazirolan D, Yalvac IS, Ozer PA, Aslan BS, Duman S. Incidence and prognosis of ocular hypertension secondary to viral uveitis. *Int Ophthalmol.* 2010;30:191-194. Epub 2009 Apr 3.

The Herpetic Eye Disease Study Group. A controlled trial of oral acyclovir for the prevention of stromal keratitis or iritis in patients with herpes simplex virus epithelial keratitis. The epithelial keratitis trial. *Arch Ophthalmol.* 1997;115:703-12. Erratum in: *Arch Ophthalmol* 1997;115:1196.

Van der Lelij A, Ooijman FM, Kijlstra A, Rothova A. Anterior uveitis with sectoral iris atrophy in the absence of keratitis: a distinct clinical entity among herpetic eye diseases. *Ophthalmology.* 2000;107:1164-1170.

Yamamoto S, Pavan-Langston D, Kinoshita S, Nishida K, Shimomura Y. Detecting herpes virus DNA in uveitis using the polymerase chain reaction. *Br J Ophthalmol.* 1996;80:465-468.

WHEN SHOULD I BE SUSPICIOUS OF
TUBERCULOSIS AND WHAT TESTING IS USEFUL?

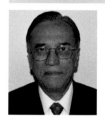

Narsing A. Rao, MD

Although ocular tuberculosis (TB) is rare in the developed world, an increase in the migration of people from regions of endemic TB has led to a re-emergence of this ocular infection in the United States and other western countries and to a re-emphasis on its recognition. The use of polymerase chain reaction (PCR) and gamma interferon release assays has helped make possible the early diagnosis of intraocular TB in both endemic and nonendemic regions of world and has helped define the clinical features of ocular TB.[1-5] In endemic and nonendemic countries, a mycobacterial ocular infection can manifest with diverse clinical features, primarily depending on the lodgment of the bacteria in the ocular or ocular adnexal structures. The route of such bacterial dissemination is usually from the lung to the eye. In more than 90% of exposed individuals, the bacteria can remain dormant in the lung or in extrapulmonary organs, including the eye. Microbial reactivation at these sites occurs at a later period, usually months to years, leading to the clinical manifestation of the infection. In the eye, however, such extrapulmonary infection usually presents in the absence of clinically apparent pulmonary or other extrapulmonary disease.[2] Of the various clinical manifestations of ocular TB, the most common presentation is an intraocular inflammation/uveitis in the form of anterior, intermediate, posterior (Figure 17-1), or panuveitis; choroidal or subretinal mass; retinal periphlebitis or vasculitis; optic neuropathy; and sclerouveitis.

In recent histologically proven cases of ocular TB, posterior and panuveitis were common in both adults and children.[3] Similarly, clinical studies suggest that the most frequent presentation of TB posterior uveitis is in the form of multifocal choroiditis, serpiginous-like choroiditis, or combined features of both in the form of multifocal serpiginoid choroiditis.[4] The latter is typically seen in regions of endemic TB and in patients who

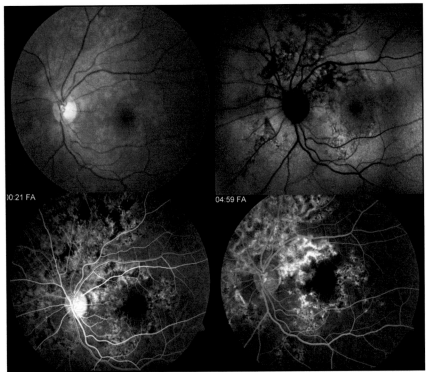

Figure 17-1. Fundus findings in a 42-year-old Asian-Indian with presumed intraocular TB. Note multifocal serpiginoid choroiditis changes that can be documented well with fundus autofluorescence (upper right) and by fluorescein angiography.

migrate from such regions. These patients, who are usually young or middle-aged, present with unilateral or bilateral vitritis and multifocal choroidal lesions with a geographic pattern distributed in the posterior pole and midperiphery of the choroid. Unlike in classic serpiginous choroiditis, the TB lesions rarely extend from the juxtapapillary choroid. The multifocal serpiginoid lesions usually reveal chorioretinal scars of geographic appearance with hyperpigmentation from retinal pigment epithelium (RPE) hyperplasia. This pigmentation usually spares the margins (see Figure 17-1). Although patients with such fundus changes show a positive skin test for purified protein derivative (PPD) and most likely a positive gamma interferon release test (Quantiferon Gold TB test), chest x-rays can be negative. Usually, these individuals respond well to anti-TB treatment with no recurrence of the ocular inflammation.[4]

The ophthalmologist should suspect a TB etiology when patients present with granulomatous uveitis, multifocal serpiginoid choroiditis, retinal periphlebitis or vasculitis, a history of previous exposure to TB, and negative clinical and laboratory features suggestive of other diagnoses. Such patients, particularly migrants from endemic TB regions, those who are HIV-positive or have other immunodeficiencies, and the elderly, require further investigation as will be outlined, or a therapeutic multidrug trial (3 or 4 agents) of anti-TB agents: isoniazid, rifampin, streptomycin, and ethambutol usually in combination with oral corticosteroids (0.5 to 1 mg/kg of body weight) in consultation with a pulmonologist with expertise in the management of pulmonary TB. Usually, such a therapeutic trial is continued for 6 to 10 weeks. A positive response requires further continuation of the treatment, and such patients are diagnosed as presumed ocular TB. If the patient does not respond to the trial of anti-TB agents, it is less likely that the ocular inflammation is from the mycobacterial infection.

Nonimmigrant native elderly individuals and HIV-positive patients can also develop intraocular TB. Elderly patients with intraocular TB show a positive PPD test, and chest x-rays may reveal scarring consistent with healed or, rarely, active pulmonary TB. In elderly patients, TB multifocal serpiginoid choroiditis can be differentiated from typical serpiginous choroiditis. The latter is characterized by minimal or no vitritis and by larger solitary lesions that extend from the juxtapapillary choroid to involve the posterior pole but usually spare the midperiphery from independent lesions. Moreover, patients with typical serpiginous choroiditis show negative chest x-ray findings and negative PPD.

The gold standard to establish a diagnosis of intraocular TB is a culture of the affected tissue, but this is rarely performed. Thus, in ophthalmic patients, the clinical diagnosis of the ocular infection remains as presumed ocular TB. The tools commonly used to support a clinical impression of ocular TB include PPD and/or gamma interferon release assay and chest x-ray.[5] The criteria for diagnosis of presumed ocular TB is based usually on the demonstration of a positive PPD, chest x-ray findings consistent with pulmonary TB (although this can be negative), and response to multi-drug anti-TB treatment. In contrast, the demonstration of mycobacteria DNA by PCR or a positive culture of the ocular fluid or tissue in uveitis is considered definitive intraocular TB/uveitis. Rare patients with uveitis may show manifestations of active pulmonary TB or lymphadenopathy with demonstrable bacteria in the sputum or in the lymph node biopsy; such cases may also be considered definitive intraocular TB. Although there have been advances in diagnostic testing, such as in-vitro gamma interferon release assay and PCR, the former cannot differentiate an active infection from latent disease. Positive PCR test results are useful, but negative results cannot rule out ocular TB. Thus, in most instances, the diagnosis of intraocular TB is made retrospectively and mainly as presumed intraocular TB.

References

1. Rao NA, Saraswathy S, Smith RE. Tuberculous uveitis: distribution of Mycobacterium tuberculosis in the retinal pigment epithelium. *Arch Ophthalmol.* 2006;124:1777-1779.
2. Gupta V, Gupta A, Rao NA. Intraocular tuberculosis—an update. *Surv Ophthalmol.* 2007;52:561-587.
3. Wroblewski KJ, Hidayat AA, Neafie RC, Rao NA, Zapor M. Ocular tuberculosis: a clinicopathologic and molecular study. *Ophthalmology.* 2011;118:772-777. Epub 2010 Nov 4.
4. Vasconcelos-Santos DV, Rao PK, Davies JB, Sohn EH, Rao NA. Clinical features of tuberculous serpiginous like choroiditis in contrast to classic serpiginous choroiditis. *Arch Ophthalmol.* 2010;128:853-858.
5. Vasconcelos-Santos DV, Zierhut M , Rao NA. Strengths and weaknesses of diagnostic tools for tuberculous uveitis. *Ocul Immunol Inflamm.* 2009;17:351-355.

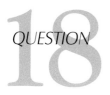

HOW OFTEN SHOULD I EXAMINE A CHILD WITH JUVENILE IDIOPATHIC ARTHRITIS?

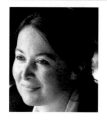

Sofia Androudi, MD
(co-authored with Evangelia Tsironi, MD and
Periklis Brazitikos, MD)

Unlike the joints, ocular involvement with juvenile rheumatoid arthritis is most often asymptomatic, yet, the inflammation can cause serious morbidity with loss of vision. Overall, the frequency varies from 2% to 34% in children with juvenile idiopathic arthritis (JIA).[1]

The onset is usually asymptomatic (in more than 50%), and therefore screening by slit-lamp is essential for diagnosis. Children with JIA remain at risk of developing uveitis into adulthood. There are reports of uveitis diagnosed initially more than 20 years after the onset of arthritis.[1] The activity of the uveal inflammation does not parallel that of the joint disease.[2] The onset of ocular inflammation is insidious and asymptomatic in most young children.[1] Because of the lack of symptoms or the cognitive recognition by the child, the exact time of onset of ocular involvement is frequently difficult to determine. This observation emphasizes the requirement for slit-lamp examination by an ophthalmologist at the diagnosis of JIA and periodically thereafter.

Early detection and treatment can prevent the development of complications and can prevent permanent visual impairment. These complications are more frequent and more severe in younger children and are often asymptomatic. The most frequent cause of avoidable morbidity remains missed or inadequate examinations[2] in the first year of disease, and all efforts must be made to achieve early and thorough examinations.

Principles

1. Initial screening examination: Uveitis often starts soon after onset of arthritis but may also start before the arthritis. The initial screening examination is therefore a clinical priority and should occur as soon as possible and no later than 6 weeks from referral rather than waiting for the first available appointment.
2. Symptomatic patients, or patients suspected of cataracts or synechiae, should be seen within a week of referral.
3. Parent information: Parents of children with JIA need to be fully informed about the possibility of uveitis and that this is usually an asymptomatic condition until complications arise. They should be instructed to seek medical assessment urgently if their child develops visual symptoms or signs such as red eyes, photophobia, abnormal pupils, corneal clouding, or visual impairment. In younger children, this may be evident by unusual blinking, eye rubbing, visual inattention or preferential attention on auditory signals, or a new onset squint.
4. Training: Ophthalmologists and other health care professionals carrying out uveitis screening should be appropriately trained and experienced. They should have facilities to audit the outcomes of their screening program. Parents must be fully informed about the method of screening and the need to attend for specific uveitis screening examinations on a regular basis. Arrangements need to be in place to give priority to rebooking of any missed appointments in this group with a system of contacting no-show appointments.
5. Older patients: Teenage patients need to be told to return quickly should they become symptomatic. If there is concern about their reliability, then they should be considered for longer-term frequent screening.
6. On stopping immunosuppressant treatment such as methotrexate: Patients who have been treated with methotrexate for their arthritis may not have developed uveitis due to drug-related immunosuppression. However, after methotrexate is stopped, uveitis may flare. Screening should therefore restart at 2-month intervals after stopping methotrexate or any other immunosuppressant therapy during the period of maximum risk for 6 months before reverting to the previous screening arrangements.

The suggested frequency of ophthalmologic visits for children with JIA without known uveitis at diagnosis and during follow-up is presented in Table 18-1. It is unclear how often children with JIA should be screened for this complication. From a review of the literature, the following recommendations can be proposed[3-5]: if uveitis is not detected initially, all children with JIA should be screened by slit-lamp examinations every 3 months for the first 5 years after arthritis onset. After 7 years, screening could be stopped. The only exceptions would be arthritic children at low risk for uveitis (eg, systemic-onset JIA; juvenile spondyloarthropathy; and juvenile onset rheumatoid arthritis, who do not need to be screened if the initial slit-lamp examination is normal). However, there may be a delay in being certain about the diagnosis or exact category of JIA, and overlaps between groups do occur.

Table 18-1
Frequency of Ophthalmologic Examination in Patients With Juvenile Idiopathic Arthritis

Type	ANA	Age at Onset, y	Duration of Disease, y	Risk Category	Eye Examination Frequency, months
Oligoarthritis or polyarthritis	+	≤6	≤4	High	3
	+	≤6	>4	Moderate	6
	+	≤6	>7	Low	12
	+	>6	≤4	Moderate	6
	+	>6	>4	Low	12
	−	≤6	≤4	Moderate	6
	−	≤6	>4	Low	12
	−	>6	NA	Low	12
Systemic disease (fever, rash)	NA	NA	NA	Low	12

ANA indicates antinuclear antibodies; NA, not applicable.
Recommendations for follow-up continue through childhood and adolescence.
Adapted from Cassidy J, Kivlin J, Lindsley C, Nocton J. Ophthalmologic examinations in children with juvenile rheumatoid arthritis. *Pediatrics.* 2006;117:1843-1845.

When patients are discharged from the regular screening program, it is vital to stress to them that they, and the family, are now deemed able to detect any changes in their vision that may signify a new onset or flare of uveitis. It does NOT mean that their risk of uveitis has gone away completely. A tip for family self-monitoring is to remind the young patient to self-check the vision (ie, by reading small print with each eye once a week). Monitoring may need to continue indefinitely if there are other reasons why the young person may be unable to detect a change in vision or may be unwilling to seek re-referral (eg, learning difficulties or treatment noncompliance).

References

1. Rosenberg IS. Uveitis associated with childhood rheumatic diseases. *Curr Opin Rheumatol.* 2002;14:542-547.
2. Cimaz RG, Fink CW. The articular prognosis of pauciarticular onset juvenile arthritis is not influenced by the presence of uveitis. *J Rheumatol.* 1996;23:357-359.
3. Southwood TR, Ryder CA. Ophthalmological screening in juvenile arthritis: should the frequency of screening be based on the risk of developing chronic iridocyclitis? *Br J Rheumatol.* 1992;31:633-634.
4. Cassidy J, Kivlin J, Lindsley C, Nocton J. Ophthalmologic examinations in children with juvenile rheumatoid arthritis. *Pediatrics.* 2006;117:1843-1845.
5. Royal College of Ophthalmologists; British Society for Pediatric and Adolescent Rheumatology. *Guidelines for Screening for Uveitis in Juvenile Idiopathic Arthritis (JIA).* London, UK: Royal College of Ophthalmologists; 2006.

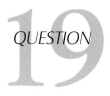

HOW SHOULD I USE TOPICAL MYDRIATIC AND CYCLOPLEGIC AGENTS?

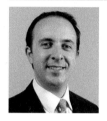

Stephen D. Anesi, MD

Topical mydriatic and cycloplegic agents are an integral part of the daily routine of eye care specialists, often used for both diagnostic and therapeutic purposes. Mydriasis is dilation of the pupil by means of dilator contraction by adrenergic agonists or sphincter relaxation by muscarinic antagonists. Cycloplegia is the paralysis of the ciliary muscle by antimuscarinics, inhibiting accommodation and decreasing tension on the scleral spur. The efficacy and length of effect produced depends on each agent, as stronger agents tend to be longer acting. Indications for use include cycloplegic refraction, dilation for ophthalmoscopy and testing, surgery, suppression during amblyopic therapy, palliative care for phthisis, and uveitis. Several examples of these medications (eg, atropine, homatropine, and cyclopentolate) actually possess both characteristics and prove to be the most relied upon agents in the treatment of uveitis.

This dual action is useful in uveitis therapy for several reasons. Ocular pain and photophobia induced by ciliary spasm can potentially be reduced. There is thought that decreased vascular permeability may lead to lower amounts of inflammatory cells and protein in the anterior chamber (flare). Most importantly, avoidance of the formation of new and severing of previously formed posterior synechiae, which can severely limit both visual acuity as well as diagnostic capabilities, is achieved during dilation by virtue of decreased contact of the posterior iris with the anterior lens capsule as well as the cycloplegic decrease in lens thickness and convexity.[1] Dark-pigmented irides are notoriously less responsive to these agents and may require increased dosing or a stronger agent.

Opinions vary widely on which agents to use and when to use them. Table 19-1 shows one such example of an algorithm for using mydriatic and cycloplegic therapy. Some treat with any evidence of anterior chamber inflammation. For mild to moderate iritis, I generally observe without use of these agents while treating the inflammation as

Table 19-1

Timing and Duration of Action of Commonly Used Cycloplegic-Mydriatic Agents

Drug	Time to Maximum Effect After Topical Application		Duration of Action After Topical Application		Indications
	Mydriasis	Cycloplegia	Mydriasis	Cycloplegia	
Atropine	30 to 40 minutes	1 day	7 to 10 days	2 weeks	Anterior uveitis Cycloplegic refraction Suppression amblyopia
Homatropine	30 to 60 minutes	30 to 60 minutes	1 to 2 days	1 to 2 days	Anterior uveitis
Cyclopentolate	15 to 30 minutes	15 to 30 minutes	24 hours	24 hours	Anterior uveitis Cycloplegic refraction Fundus photography and ophthalmoscopy
Tropicamide	15 to 30 minutes	25 minutes	4 to 6 hours	6 hours	Fundus photography and ophthalmoscopy

Adapted from Titcomb LC. Mydriatic-cycloplegic drugs and corticosteroids. *Pharmaceutical Journal.* 1999;263: 900-905.

necessary. Extreme symptoms of photophobia or more severe or stubborn inflammation may eventually prompt the temporary addition of a cycloplegic, especially with signs of impending synechiae. The most popular treatment options include cyclopentolate 1% and homatropine 2%. Each has sufficient cycloplegic efficacy along with an intermediate length of action (24 hours or more) and can be dosed 2 to 4 times daily until the inflammation recedes. Cyclopentolate may have a disadvantage as it has been shown to be a chemoattractant to inflammatory cells in vitro.[2] A short-acting agent such as tropicamide 1% is useful for diagnostic purposes, and it is arguable that a 4-times-daily dosing schedule may allow sufficient mobility of the iris to prevent synechiae, but this would likely be at the expense of poorly reducing symptoms as it is only weakly cycloplegic.

The reverse argument can be made for atropine 1%, a more powerful and longer-acting cycloplegic, which may allow for greater control of ciliary spasm and prevention of central synechiae. Its potency, however, effectively immobilizes the iris for days at a time and, while not allowing mobility, could conceivably contribute to synechiae in the dilated state. Additionally, atropine has a lasting effect on visual acuity, and potential systemic side effects are problematic. Scopolamine 0.25% may have a cycloplegic efficacy similar to atropine and a shorter duration of effect, but it unfortunately has a greater ability to cross the blood-brain barrier and affect central nervous system receptors.

A so-called "dynamite cocktail" of potent agents (ie, atropine 1%, epinephrine 1:1000, and cocaine 4%) in concert with a cotton pledget may be employed when synechiolysis is particularly difficult.[3] Subconjunctival injection of a combination of atropine, procaine, and adrenaline has also been used, but with serious potential systemic effects.[4] Sympathetic agonists such as phenylephrine 10%, while not helpful with cycloplegia, are effective mydriatics and can be used to aid synechiolysis. Phenylephrine 10% has been shown to induce the release of pigment granules into the anterior chamber, possibly through pigment epithelial degeneration during iris contraction, which, though microscopically distinct, can easily be misinterpreted as inflammation or microhyphema in the appropriate setting. Proper evaluation of the anterior chamber should always be performed prior to application of any mydriatic when looking for cell and flare.

Disadvantages of these agents include the severe stinging many patients experience upon application that can sometimes be more bothersome than the ciliary spasm it was intended to treat. Patients are relieved upon discontinuation not only for this reason, but because of the significant blurring created by cycloplegia. An endpoint in cycloplegic treatment must be considered in every case. There should almost never be a reason to submit to standing doses of these cycloplegic agents. Still, significant active uveitis must always be addressed with aggressive treatment until it is quiet, and it may be reasonable to use these agents for long periods when all efforts to squelch the fire are being thwarted. Along with blurring and the general discomfort produced, ocular side effects include atopic response to the medication or vehicle, which may affect the lids or the ocular surface. Multiple medications and confusion in dosage may increase risk of noncompliance with other more vital therapy. There is also the known danger of mydriatic induction of acute closed-angle glaucoma. Interestingly, intraocular pressure in open-angle glaucoma has also been shown to increase with these drops by a mechanism that is not completely understood. It is thought this may relate to trabecular outflow and the effect of changing tension on the scleral spur. One must be mindful of glaucomatocyclitic crisis, an inflammatory condition where high pressures may possibly be exacerbated by use of these agents.

Systemic side effects have also been well documented. Phenylephrine 10% may greatly increase blood pressure in infants, diabetics, and the elderly and, therefore, is usually avoided in these patients. Circulating levels of cycloplegics may exert an effect on muscarinic receptors throughout the body, initially causing dry mouth and flushing. Other more serious documented effects include urinary retention, tachycardia, somnolence, ataxia, hallucinations, and seizures. There have even been reports of abuse of and dependence on cyclopentolate.[5] These are rare and generally stem from overuse of the stronger drops like atropine; however, some severe effects have also been seen with therapeutic levels of even weak cycloplegics. Again, infants and the elderly seem especially prone to this, as well as White males with Down syndrome, and care of these patients should reflect this.

Mydriatic-cycloplegic agents have their place in the treatment of uveitis. Whether they should be used and in what circumstances are up for debate. I suggest they be treated similar to topical steroids in that they may occasionally be used for acute symptoms and rescue (from synechiae), but that they should be discontinued whenever possible.

References

1. Bartlett JD, Jaanus SD, eds. *Clinical Ocular Pharmacology.* 3rd ed. Boston, MA: Butterworth-Heinemann; 1995.
2. Tsai E, Till GO, Marak GE Jr. Effects of mydriatic agents on neutrophil migration. *Ophthalmic Research.* 1988;20:14-19.
3. Foster CS, Vitale AT. *Diagnosis and Treatment of Uveitis.* Philadelphia, PA: WB Saunders Co; 2002:159-165.
4. Jayamanne DGR, Fitt AWD, Wariyer R, Cottrell DG. Persistent tachycardia following subconjunctival injections of mydriatic agents (Mydricaine) used for maintenance of perioperative mydriasis in vitreoretinal surgery. *Eye.* 1995;9:530-531.
5. Sato EH, De Frietas D, Foster CS. Abuse of cyclopentolate hydrochloride (Cyclogyl) drops. *N Engl J Med.* 1992;326:1363-1364.

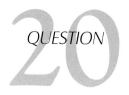

QUESTION

WHAT ARE THE INDICATIONS AND CONTRAINDICATIONS FOR THE USE OF PERIOCULAR CORTICOSTEROID INJECTIONS?

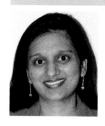

Arusha Gupta, MD
(co-authored with Esen K. Akpek, MD)

Periocular corticosteroid injection is an effective technique for treating inflammatory ocular disorders without inducing systemic side effects. This mode of delivery is generally indicated in patients who have failed hourly topical steroids, those with unilateral disease and requiring chronic treatment, and sometimes before the initiation of systemic steroids or as an adjunct to it.[1] Because the medication is administered locally, it acts as a depot, and the systemic side effects are minimal.

Commonly, there are 2 different routes of administration. Sub-Tenon's injection is a technique where a long 25-gauge needle is inserted along the surface of the eyeball superotemporally after the application of a pledget of topical anesthetic. A "sweeping" motion is made with the needle after penetration into Tenon's space in order to demonstrate that the globe has not been impaled on the tip of the needle. Another technique is "peribulbar" injection with a short 30-gauge needle through the periorbital septum just superior to the inferior orbital rim. Elevating the globe slightly with the nondominant index finger and also making a small "sweeping" motion after penetration of the septum should be performed to ensure that the sclera or globe has not been impaled on the tip of the 30-gauge needle.

Methylprednisolone acetate and triamcinolone acetonide are the 2 most commonly used preparations for these injections. Triamcinolone acetonide comes in 10 and 40 mg/mL suspension with the trade names of Kenalog and Kenalog-40, respectively. Methylprednisolone acetate comes in 80 and 160 mg/mL depot suspension with the trade name of Depo-Medrol. A small amount of local anesthetic can also be administrated in the same syringe to help with the pain.

Our preference is peribulbar injections due to safety and patient comfort. We use 40 mg of triamcinolone acetonide mixed with 0.5 mL of 2% lidocaine without epinephrine. The effect usually lasts 6 to 12 weeks. Patients with chronic inflammation often require repeated injections.

Indications

- Anterior uveitis: Periocular corticosteroid injections are indicated in cases of anterior uveitis (where inflammation is confined mostly to the anterior chamber) where hourly topical treatment has not resulted in improvement of inflammation within several days or when there is associated cystoid macular edema or high risk of developing cystoid macular edema. Some of the noninfectious causes of anterior uveitis that would respond to periocular steroids include human leukocyte antigen (HLA)-B27-related anterior uveitis,[1] uveitis associated with sero-negative arthropathies (ankylosing spondylitis, psoriatic arthritis, Reiter syndrome), and inflammatory bowel disease.

- Intermediate uveitis: In cases where inflammation is mostly involving the vitreous and ciliary body with some anterior chamber inflammation, particularly in younger patients where avoidance of systemic treatment is preferable, periocular corticosteroid injection is our first line of treatment. Some of the noninfectious causes of intermediate uveitis that would respond to periocular corticosteroids include pars planitis, uveitis associated with multiple sclerosis, and sarcoidosis.[2]

Macular edema secondary to retinal vein occlusion, diabetes, or postcataract surgery can also be treated by periocular corticosteroid injections.

Adverse Effects

Increase in intraocular pressure is the most common complication of periocular corticosteroid injections. Studies have shown that as many as 30% of eyes develop high intraocular pressure requiring chronic topical medications and up to 25% of those require glaucoma surgery to control the intraocular pressure.[1,3] Other side effects include formation of cataracts, aponeurotic ptosis, allergic reactions with conjunctival breakdown, scleral melt, endophthalmitis, peribulbar or retrobulbar hemorrhage, and of course possible globe perforation. Repeated injections may also cause orbital scarring and eventually enophthalmos.

Contraindications

Prior to starting therapy, malignancy and infectious etiologies of uveitis such as syphilis, Lyme disease, toxoplasmosis, herpetic infections, tuberculosis, and masquerade syndromes such as intraocular lymphoma must be ruled out. Caution must be taken in patients with previous history of intraocular pressure rise with topical steroids. Injections should be deferred in patients with pre-existing glaucoma with a history of steroid-induced eye pressure elevation unless glaucoma surgery is being planned in the near future. Caution must also be taken in patients with known connective tissue diseases, such as rheumatic diseases, and in patients with prior episodes of scleritis because of the possibility of scleral melts.

References

1. Lafranco Dafflon M, Tran VT, Guex-Crosier Y, Herbort CP. Posterior sub-Tenon's steroid injections for the treatment of posterior ocular inflammation: indications, efficacy and side effects. *Graefes Arch Clin Exp Ophthalmol.* 1999;237:289-295.
2. Babu BM, Rathinam SR. Intermediate uveitis. *Indian J Ophthalmol.* 2010;58:21-27.
3. Levin DS, Han DP, Dev S, et al. Subtenon's depot corticosteroid injections in patients with a history of corticosteroid-induced intraocular pressure elevation. *Am J Ophthalmol.* 2002;133:196-202.

WHEN SHOULD I SUSPECT AND HOW CAN I TELL IF MY PATIENT WITH UVEITIS HAS A MASQUERADE SYNDROME RATHER THAN AUTOIMMUNE UVEITIS?

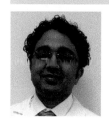

Annal Dhananjayan Meleth, MD, MS
(co authored with H. Nida Sen, MD, MHSc and
Chi-Chao Chan, MD)

Deciding when ocular inflammation is secondary to a neoplastic or infectious cause requires a high index of suspicion and a thorough clinical evaluation. An infectious cause for uveitis should be ruled out prior to beginning immunosuppressive therapy for a patient with autoimmune uveitis. The clinical history and social history can be quite helpful. It is essential to rule out 2 of the great infectious masqueraders in medicine: syphilis and tuberculosis (TB).[1] The patients' birthplace and work history may put them at greater or lesser risk of TB (ie, a prison guard from South Asia whose mother was treated for TB is going to cause more flags to be raised than a young man from Sweden without TB exposure). Similarly, a history of high-risk behavior such as IV drug use or previous treatment for a sexually transmitted disease should raise the suspicion for syphilis. We obtain both a tuberculosis skin test (PPD) and a treponemal (FTA-ABS, MHA-TP, TPPA) along with a nontreponemal test (RPR) on all uveitis patients, as these are both treatable and potentially curable causes of uveitis. Additional aspects of the social history that may provide insight into the potential for an infectious etiology for the patients' uveitis include a travel history to endemic areas, whether the patient has any pets at home, and a history of exposures via hobbies such as hiking or fishing. The patients' medical history can also provide important clues to the patients' overall risk for an infectious etiology; immunosuppressed or immunocompromised patients require a higher index of suspicion than immunocompetent patients.

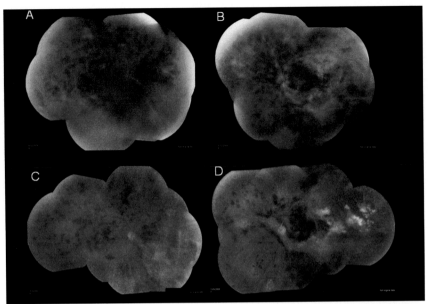

Figure 21-1. A 61-year-old man presented with a history of systemic lymphoma and a clinical appearance of bilateral central retinal vein occlusions with areas of retinitis as seen in (A) and (B). His vision was 20/250 OD and HM OS. The differential at presentation included lymphomatous infiltrates and infectious etiologies in addition to hypercoagulability secondary to the lymphoma. Due to the unusual appearance and severity of disease on presentation, a diagnostic vitreous tap was performed, which showed >250,000 cytomegalovirus PCR and no atypical lymphocytes. Aggressive therapy was instituted with intravitreal gancyclovir and foscarnet, in addition to oral valgancyclovir. Two months later, his vision had improved to 20/100 OD and 20/250 OS with a better fundus appearance as shown in (C) and (D).

The clinical exam is helpful in elucidating an infectious cause for a patients' uveitis (Figure 21-1). A unilateral anterior uveitis with concurrent iris atrophy or a unilateral retinitis that is rapidly progressive and characterized by vascular occlusive disease may lead us to suspect *Herpesviridae*. Of course, this does not mean that bilateral cases of herpetic retinitis do not occur, as acute retinal necrosis can be bilateral in up to one-third of cases and cytomegalovirus retinitis often affects both eyes. Similarly, a neuroretinitis with a positive history of cat exposure or an intermediate uveitis with a history of tick bites may raise the index of suspicion for *Bartonella* infection or Lyme disease, respectively. Patients with infectious uveitis may manifest a worsening of disease while on immunomodulatory therapy. So, when in doubt, close follow-up can be a life saver.

Masquerade syndromes secondary to neoplasm can also be a very challenging diagnosis to make.[2] Again, the clinical history can be of paramount importance. A previous history of malignancy or AIDS or change in mental status can raise the suspicion for a metastatic malignancy or for primary intraocular (retinal) or central nervous system lymphoma. The age of the patient is helpful, as the typical patient with intraocular lymphoma is between the ages of 50 and 70 years. A history of initial improvement with anti-inflammatory therapy with subsequent recrudescence of disease can also be an important clue to a neoplastic process.

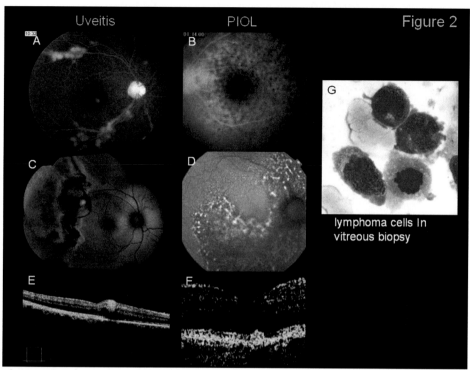

Figure 21-2. (A, C, and E) Imaging modalities demonstrating differences between an autoimmune uveitis and (B, D, and F) a PIOL. (B) Fluorescein angiography demonstrates the characteristic "leopard spot" appearance, (C) while fundus autofluorescence shows diffuse mottling in the setting of intraocular lymphoma. (F) OCT imaging shows a lesion in the deep retina in the setting of lymphoma. (G) Vitreous sampling illustrates malignant cells with an elevated IL-10 to IL-6 ratio.

On clinical exam, a vitritis with sheets and clumps of vitreous cells but little haze can increase the suspicion for primary intraocular lymphoma (PIOL). Uveal involvement is more likely in the setting of metastasis while PIOL has a predilection for the retina, retinal pigment epithelium (RPE), and optic nerve. Fluorescein angiography can demonstrate a leopard spot appearance, fundus autofluorescence imaging can show diffuse RPE involvement and mottled signal, and optical coherence tomography (OCT) imaging may demonstrate the lesions at the RPE level (Figure 21-2). To confirm a clinical suspicion of a neoplastic process, we prefer sampling of ocular fluid, ideally vitreous, via diagnostic vitrectomy or aspiration. We find cytological and cytokine analysis quite useful. A greater than 1.0 ratio of vitreal interleukin-10 to interleukin-6 is suspicious for B-cell lymphoma in our lab.[2,3] Multiple vitreous biopsies may be required to identify malignant cells, as they are easily necrotic, admix with reactive lymphocytes, and are sensitive to corticosteroid therapy and mishandling. A chorioretinal biopsy by an experienced vitreoretinal surgeon with subsequent histopathological examination by an ophthalmic pathologist can also provide valuable information. A systemic evaluation is required for patients in whom a neoplastic etiology is suspected. Patients with a suspicion for intraocular lymphoma warrant central nervous system (CNS) imaging and lumbar puncture with cytology on the cerebrospinal fluid. If a patient has already been demonstrated to have neoplastic cells in the cerebrospinal fluid, a vitreous biopsy is not needed in the setting of appropriate clinical findings. Patients in whom metastatic disease is suspected should be referred to a neuro-oncologist or hemato-oncologist.

Summary

A thorough history and a careful ocular examination including systemic and ocular imaging are the key to differentiating an infectious or neoplastic etiology to autoimmune uveitis. A few important points to keep in mind: if the uveitis looks atypical for the age, ethnicity, and gender of the patient or if it fails to improve or gets worse on anti-inflammatory therapy, you must continue your skepticism and further work-up to rule out infection or malignancy.

Acknowledgment

The National Eye Institute Intramural Research Program funded the study.

References

1. Whitcup SM, Nussenblatt R. *Fundamentals and Clinical Practice: Expert Consult, Uveitis.* 4th ed. Philadelphia, PA: Mosby; 2010.
2. Chan CC, Gonzales JA. *Primary Intraocular Lymphoma.* Hackensack, NJ: World Scientific Publishing Co; 2007.
3. Buggage RR, Whitcup SM, Nussenblatt RB, Chan CC. Using interleukin-10 to interleukin-6 ratio to distinguish primary intraocular lymphoma and uveitis. *Invest Ophthalmol Vis Sci.* 1999;40:2462-2463.

The opinions expressed in this chapter are those solely of the authors and do not represent the views or official policies of the National Eye Institute or the United States National Institutes of Health.

22

HOW DO I TREAT CYTOMEGALOVIRUS RETINITIS IN A PATIENT WITH AIDS?

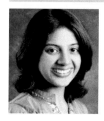

Sana S. Siddique, MD
(co-authored with Muhammad Kashif Israr, MBBS)

Cytomegalovirus (CMV) retinitis is the most common ocular manifestation of the acquired immunodeficiency syndrome (AIDS), accounting for 40% of visual loss to 20/200 or worse in such patients. The associated risks of CMV retinitis include immune recovery retinitis and retinal detachment.[1,2]

Initial Therapy

Ganciclovir, cidofovir, and foscarnet are all intravenously-administered drugs for CMV retinitis and are now largely replaced by valganciclovir (approved in 2001) in oral form with almost the same bioavailability as intravenous ganciclovir.

The choice of initial treatment depends on the location and extent of the lesion, as well as the level of immune suppression, renal status, concomitant drugs, adherence to anti-retroviral therapy (ART), and lifestyle considerations.[2]

In the case of newly diagnosed CMV retinitis, the key step in initial therapy is to commence highly active antiretroviral therapy (HAART), in order to establish immune recovery followed by anti-CMV therapy.[2]

Oral valganciclovir at a dose of 900 mg twice daily for 21 days is the preferred initial therapy for small peripheral lesions followed by a maintenance dose of 900 mg once daily. This regimen arrests CMV progression in more than 90% of eyes and achieves satisfactory clinical response in 72% of patients.[3] If the lesion is sight-threatening (ie, adjacent to the optic nerve or less than 1500 µm from fovea), then a combination of ganciclovir implant followed by oral valganciclovir is the preferred choice over daily intravenous ganciclovir.[2] Studies comparing ganciclovir implant with intravenous ganciclovir as

Table 22-1
Summary of the Available Systemic Anti-Cytomegalovirus Drugs

Antiviral Drug	Induction	Maintenance	Advantages	Side Effects
Ganciclovir	IV: 5 mg/kg BID for 2 to 3 weeks Implant: 4.5 mg 5 to 8 months	IV: 5 mg/kg QD	Implant: Long time to retinitis progression	Bone marrow suppression: Intraocular implant related.
Foscarnet	60 mg/kg TID for 2 to 3 weeks	30 to 40 mg/kg TID	Anti-HIV activity	Nephrotoxicity
Cidofovir	IV: 5 mg/kg for 2 weeks	IV: 5 mg/kg for 2 weeks	Least expensive, infrequent dosing	Nephrotoxicity and uveitis
Valganciclovir	PO: 900 mg BID for 3 weeks	PO: 900 mg QD	Per oral, QD dose	Bone marrow suppression

IV indicates intravenous; BID, twice a day; TID, 3 times a day; PO, by mouth; QD, once a day; HIV, human immunodeficiency virus.

initial therapy for CMV retinitis have shown the risk of progression to be 3 times more in intravenous ganciclovir-treated patients; however, the ganciclovir implant alone in the absence of any systemic therapy was associated with contralateral retinitis and extraocular CMV complications.[1,2]

Cidofovir, though much more potent than other anti-CMV drugs, is rarely used due to the requirement for intermittent intravenous administration and dose-dependent, irreversible nephrotoxicity (Table 22-1).

Foscarnet is another potent drug that has been used as initial therapy. It is highly nephrotoxic and has to be intravenously administered; therefore, its use is limited, and it is mainly used as a second-line therapy in cases of resistance to ganciclovir or dose-limiting neutropenia.[3] Intravitreal foscarnet has been used in the past and was shown to be associated with recurrence of the retinitis (33.3%) within 20 weeks.[3]

Discontinuation of Anti-Cytomegalovirus Therapy

Discontinuing anti-CMV therapy can be considered after the immune system has recovered with HAART. The most important parameters to assess, before discontinuing the therapy, are a sustained rise in CD4+ T-lymphocyte count (ie, 100 to 150 cells/uL) or a drop in human immunodeficiency virus (HIV) blood level and the inactivity of CMV retinitis lesions.[1,2]

Monitoring

Patients have to be regularly followed on a monthly basis with dilated fundus examination to prevent relapse and to monitor for adverse effects. The aim of systemic therapy should be to treat both the infected eye as well as to prevent recurrence in the contralateral eye.

Immune recovery uveitis (IRU) is an immune reaction to the CMV antigen by the immune system manifested as anterior uveitis, vitritis, epiretinal membrane, or macular edema. IRU is usually treated with oral/parenteral or periocular steroids, but there are no significant data available on the comparison of oral to periocular steroids. Intravitreal triamcinolone acetonide may be more effective, especially to treat macular edema, but repeated injections are required.[2]

Adverse effects associated with ganciclovir include neutropenia, thrombocytopenia, nausea and vomiting, and renal impairment. Foscarnet is associated with nephrotoxicity, anemia, and electrolyte imbalance, while the main adverse effect of cidofovir is irreversible nephrotoxicity.

Treatment Failure

Poor intraocular penetration of the systemic drugs can cause early treatment failure and is usually treated with placement of a ganciclovir implant. Drug resistance, although much less common in the HAART era, often causes late treatment failure. Mutations in CMV UL 97 and CMV UL 54 genes are responsible for low- and high-level resistance to ganciclovir, respectively. Cross-resistance to cidofovir and foscarnet is also common in such cases.[1-3]

Treatment During Pregnancy

The indication for CMV treatment in pregnant women is the same as nonpregnant HIV-infected women. Intraocular implant or intravitreous injection should be used in the first trimester to prevent fetal exposure to systemic antiviral drugs. Animal studies have shown ganciclovir, foscarnet, and cidofovir to be teratogenic and embryotoxic. On the basis of limited data, valganciclovir is considered the drug of choice in pregnancy; however, regular monitoring by fetal ultrasound and periodic fetal-movement charting is necessary.

References

1. Kaplan JE, Benson C, Holmes KH, et al. Guidelines for prevention and treatment of opportunistic infections in HIV-infected adults and adolescents: recommendations from CDC, the National Institutes of Health, and the HIV Medicine Association of the Infectious Diseases Society of America. *MMWR Recomm Rep.* 2009;58:1.
2. Holland GN. AIDS and ophthalmology: the first quarter century. *Am J Ophthalmol.* 2008;145:397.
3. Stewart MW. Optimal management of cytomegalovirus retinitis in patients with AIDS. *Clinical Ophthalmology.* 2010;26:285-299.

WHAT ARE THE CAUSES OF KERATOUVEITIS?

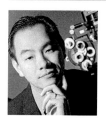

David S. Chu, MD

Keratouveitis is an inflammatory condition of the eyes characterized by keratitis and anterior uveitis. Causes of keratouveitis include viral and other infections, autoimmunity, and reaction to various exogenous agents. Viral etiology is the most common cause. However, there are numerous case reports in the literature of varied exogenous-inciting agents of keratouveitis suggesting that any potential inflammatory agent applied to the cornea can result in the local inflammation characteristic of keratouveitis. Therefore, careful history taking is essential in deciphering the etiology in patients with keratouveitis.

Keratouveitis presents with variable symptoms commonly associated with other ocular inflammatory diseases. Patients with keratouveitis may experience visual disturbance, photophobia, red eyes, tearing, or pain and discomfort. In some cases, the pain and discomfort may seem less than the findings would indicate. On examination, the degree of inflammation can also vary among patients. Keratitis can occur in any layer of the cornea: epithelium, stroma, or endothelium. The anterior chamber reaction varies in degree and can be either granulomatous or nongranulomatous. Keratouveitis is associated with cataract formation, synechiae formation, glaucoma, and corneal endothelial cell loss. Keratouveitis is sometimes recurrent. Long-term and permanent visual loss is a serious consequence of keratouveitis.

Viral Etiologies

Herpes simplex virus type 1 (HSV type 1) is the most common cause of keratouveitis in the United States (Figure 23-1); however, HSV type 2 and herpes zoster virus (HZV) are also possible viral causes. Inflammation typically presents unilaterally and can be recurrent in the same eye. The diagnosis is often established on clinical appearance and findings. Both keratitis and uveitis can present over a wide range. Keratitis can present

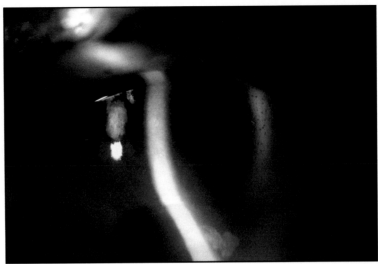

Figure 23-1. Herpes simplex keratouveitis with keratic precipitates and iritis.

as epitheliitis, stromal keratitis, sectoral keratitis, interstitial keratitis, or well-demarcated endotheliitis with corneal edema. Patients may also present with decreased corneal sensation in the ipsilateral eye. If needed, aqueous and/or corneal specimens may be obtained for viral culture or polymerase chain reaction (PCR) analysis.

Cytomegalovirus (CMV) has also been known to cause keratouveitis. Aqueous specimens have shown the presence of CMV DNA in certain patients with keratouveitis based on PCR analysis. CMV may be an under-recognized etiology of keratouveitis.[1]

Epstein-Barr virus (EBV) has been associated with stromal keratitis and anterior uveitis.

Other Causes

Tuberculosis, syphilis, Lyme disease, and leprosy are also known infectious etiologies of keratouveitis. Unlike HSV and HZV, these etiologies present bilaterally. Careful history taking and physical examination of the whole body may reveal important clues that can help with establishing proper diagnosis.

Autoimmune keratitis may be seen in patients with systemic autoimmune diseases, such as systemic lupus erythematosus, Cogan syndrome, or sarcoidosis. These conditions are known to cause keratitis or anterior uveitis; however, the clinical appearance in these cases is usually different from disease of viral etiology. Sarcoidosis can present with posterior corneal thickening, which is likely a manifestation of inflammation, or interstitial keratitis along with uveitis.

Given the immunologically and anatomically unique nature of the eye, various other agents that can come into contact with the cornea have the potential to incite ocular inflammation. There are numerous reports of various other agents that cause keratouveitis. One example is euphorbia plants, which secrete a toxic, milky-colored sap that is irritating to ocular surfaces. Cases of keratouveitis following exposure have been reported.[2]

Another example, spider keratouveitis, has also been reported in the literature.[3] Some species of arachnids, such as tarantulas, are capable of releasing bristle-like hairs from their bodies as a self-defense mechanism. I once treated a pet shop employee who was handling a tarantula when it launched hundreds, if not thousands, of these microscopic hairs into his face. The hairs I found on the corneal surface were removed; however, many more were deeply embedded in the cornea and resulted in keratitis. Over the following year, these embedded hairs migrated out of the cornea, either to the outer surface—at which time I removed them—or into the anterior chamber. When they reached the anterior chamber, keratic precipitate and anterior uveitis developed; however, the inflammation was readily controlled with topical corticosteroids.

Summary

Keratouveitis is intraocular inflammation presenting in the cornea and anterior chamber with a wide range of presentations. The possible etiology spans a wide spectrum; however, herpes virus is the most common cause. Careful history taking as well as complete physical examination may reveal potential causative agents.

References

1. Anshu A, Chee SP, Mehta JS, Tan DT. Cytomegalovirus endotheliitis in Descemet's stripping endothelial keratoplasty. *Ophthalmology*. 2009;116:624-630.
2. Scott IU, Karp CL. Euphorbia sap keratopathy: four cases and a possible pathogenic mechanism. *Br J Ophthalmol*. 1996;80:823-826.
3. Watts P, Mcpherson R, Hawksworth NR. Tarantula keratouveitis. *Cornea*. 2000;19:393-394.

WHICH MEDICATIONS CAN INDUCE UVEITIS?

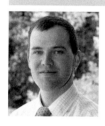

Nicholas J. Butler, MD
(co-authored with Eric B. Suhler, MD, MPH)

As with all uveitides of any cause, patients with drug-induced uveitis may complain of redness, eye pain, blurry vision, and photophobia. The consulted ophthalmologist may observe, in addition to findings corroborating the above, corneal edema, keratic precipitates (granulomatous or nongranulomatous), intraocular pressure disturbances, cell and flare, synechiae, and vitritis. As such, a careful review of medications, with particular attention to those recently prescribed, must be performed for all patients with newly diagnosed uveitis.

A review of the literature for case reports and series, in addition to postmarketing surveillance registries such as the National Registry of Drug-Induced Ocular Side Effects and those of the Food and Drug Administration (FDA), will yield more than 100 associations between prescribed and over-the-counter medications and uveitis.[1] Several routes of administration—systemic, topical, periocular, intravitreal, and intracameral—have been implicated, though the specific mechanisms for induction of uveitis are rarely, if ever, known. We will review in more detail the more common and/or clinically relevant associations here.

Bisphosphonates, commonly employed in the treatment of osteoporosis and malignant or dystrophic diseases involving the skeletal system, have been associated with uveitis, nonspecific conjunctivitis, episcleritis, and scleritis. The majority of cases have been linked to pamidronate disodium; however, alendronate sodium and others in the class have also been implicated.[1] With timely institution of topical steroids for uveitis, therapy may often be continued; however, scleritis typically resolves only with stoppage of the offending bisphosphonate.[1]

Several antibiotics have been causally linked to uveitis, most notably rifabutin, sulfonamides, and fluoroquinolones. Rifabutin, most commonly employed in the treatment of mycobacterial infections, causes uveitis in nearly 40% of treated subjects, after a mean of 65 days of treatment.[1] The classically associated hypopyon develops in a minority. The mechanism may involve a reaction to killed mycobacteria within iris tissue.[1] The uveitis generally responds readily to topical steroids, whether the rifabutin is continued, stopped, or reduced in dosage. Sulfonamide-associated uveitis develops much faster, often as early as 8 days.[1] Given the plethora of effective alternatives, antibiotic substitution is generally advised. Moxifloxacin, a fluoroquinolone with broad-spectrum antibacterial activity, has newly been linked to a uveitis-like syndrome with iris transillumination defects.[2] In our clinic at the Casey Eye Institute, we recently treated a woman with levofloxacin-related anterior uveitis, vitritis, macular edema, and posterior pole drusenoid-like lesions. Her vision returned to baseline (from 20/400 to 20/40 OU), and her inflammation resolved, including the drusenoid infiltrates, with oral prednisone.

Other associations between anti-infectives and uveitis exist. Perhaps the most well known of these is the antiviral cidofovir, an acyclic nucleotide analogue indicated for cytomegalovirus retinitis infections in patients with AIDS. Between 26% and 59% of those treated with intravenous cidofovir develop a dose-dependent anterior uveitis, mostly nongranulomatous.[3] Hypotony, likely from direct ciliary body toxicity, may be a complicating issue, especially with intravitreal usage. The uveitis appears to be associated with rising CD4+ T-lymphocyte counts.[3] Although hypotony necessitates discontinuation of the drug, most cases of uveitis may be managed with topical steroids and cycloplegics. In the modern age of highly active antiretroviral therapy (HAART), cidofovir use is uncommon, and this complication is quite rarely seen. Diethylcarbamazine, an antifilarial with activity against *Onchocerca volvulus* ("river blindness") and *Loa loa*, has similarly been linked to severe iritis in topical and oral formulation. The mechanism, similar to that proposed for rifabutin, may involve an immune-mediated reaction to dead filariae as seen with the Jarisch-Herxheimer reaction.[1]

There are numerous reports relating uveitis to several vaccines, including Bacillus Calmette-Guerin (BCG); measles, mumps, rubella (MMR); diphtheria, tetanus, and pertussis (DTaP); influenza; varicella; and smallpox. More recently, evidence linking hepatitis B vaccine with uveitis has been reported.[4] The uveitis, though rare, is often fulminant, with a mean onset of 3 days post-exposure. The myriad proposed mechanisms—delayed-type hypersensitivity, deposition of immune complexes leading to complement activation, a reaction to the vaccine carrier—reflects our general lack of understanding regarding drug-induced uveitis and its potential etiologies.[4]

The association between topical glaucoma medications and uveitis, most notably beta-blockers, brimonidine, and the prostaglandin analogues, should routinely be suspected, given the ubiquitous use of these agents among our patients. In 1991, metipranolol was withdrawn from the market in the United Kingdom, given the alarming number of reports of granulomatous anterior uveitis.[1] Timolol and betaxolol, though far less commonly, have also been shown to cause anterior uveitis.[1] Treatment, in addition to often requiring discontinuation of the beta-blocker, may require 4 to 6 weeks of topical corticosteroids. Prostaglandins are by design structurally homologous to an inflammatory mediator and have been commonly reported to potentially exacerbate anterior uveitis and cystoid macular edema. However, in our experience, these drugs are usually well tolerated in uveitic patients, and we commonly employ them as a last resort in uveitic patients with refractory pressure elevation prior to proceeding with outflow surgery.

Prompt referral to an ophthalmologist, in all patients with suspected drug-induced uveitis, is vitally important, as visually significant sequelae—cataract, glaucoma, cystoid macular edema, papillitis—may rapidly ensue. Proper treatment involves early diagnosis, discontinuation of the offending medication when possible, and local (rarely oral) corticosteroids. Timely resolution should follow. If not, alternative etiologies must be considered, as uveitis frequently portends systemic disease.

References

1. Fraunfelder FW. Drug-induced ocular inflammatory diseases. *Drugs Today (Barcelona)*. 2007;43:117-123.
2. Wefers Bettink-Remeijer M, Brouwers K, van Langenhove L, et al. Uveitis-like syndrome and iris transillumination after the use of oral moxifloxacin. *Eye (London)*. 2009;23:2260-2262.
3. Ambati J, Wynne KB, Angerame MC, Robinson MR. Anterior uveitis associated with intravenous cidofovir use in patients with cytomegalovirus retinitis. *Br J Ophthalmol*. 1999;83:1153-1158.
4. Fraunfelder FW, Suhler EB, Fraunfelder FT. Hepatitis B vaccine and uveitis: an emerging hypothesis suggested by review of 32 case reports. *Cutan Ocul Toxicol*. 2010;29:26-29.

25

How Do I Diagnose and Treat
Fuchs' Heterochromic Iridocyclitis?

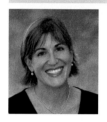

Debra A. Goldstein, MD, FRCSC

Fuchs' heterochromic iridocyclitis (FHI) is an interesting condition with fairly distinctive clinical features. It is unilateral in the majority of cases and has characteristic keratic precipitates, early-onset cataract, vitreous cells and strands, an absence of anterior and posterior synechiae, and, in most cases, no fundus pathology.

Iris heterochromia, although part of the condition's current name, is not always present. Gross inspection with diffuse white lighting, preferably sunlight, is the most reliable method of observing heterochromia. Because few of us have access to sunlight in our offices, turning the room lights on for external inspection is helpful. Careful slit-lamp examination of the iris will usually reveal atrophy, with loss of anterior stromal details and blunting of iris crypts (Figure 25-1). The amount of iris heterochromia varies considerably and is usually more obvious in White than in Black or Asian patients. Heterochromia may also not be obvious in bilateral cases in which the degree of iris change is similar. Generally speaking, the iris color of the involved eye is darker (more blue) in blue-eyed patients, whereas in brown-eyed patients, the iris color is lighter in the involved eye. Unlike the heterochromia of congenital Horner's syndrome, which is present from birth, the heterochromia of FHI is acquired. Iris nodules are sometimes seen in this condition, particularly in patients with dark irides (Figure 25-2).[1]

Gonioscopy of patients with FHI reveals an open angle, and there are often characteristic bridging vessels in the angle that do not result in angle closure; however, they may bleed during anterior chamber paracentesis (Amsler sign) or at the time of cataract surgery.

As the name implies, patients with FHI have cells in the anterior chamber and anterior vitreous. I do not believe that it ever presents as a pure iritis, and I would question the diagnosis in a patient without retrolental cells.

Figure 25-1. Anterior iris stromal atrophy in a patient with Fuchs' iridocyclitis. Note the loss of normal iris architecture and the visible iris vessels.

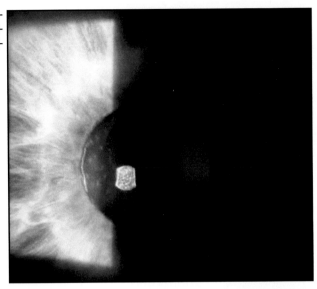

Figure 25-2. Small iris nodules are seen in this patient with FHI. Note also the characteristic KPs.

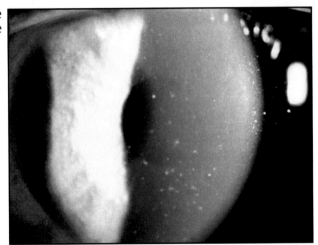

The keratic precipitates (KPs) of FHI are very characteristic. They are typically small and white and evenly distributed throughout the cornea rather than limited to Arlt's triangle. They are classically stellate in appearance, with fine extending fibrin bridges or arms (see Figures 25-2 and 25-3). Occasionally, patients with FHI will have larger, rounder KPs, but these also tend to be present throughout the whole cornea, rather than just inferiorly.

The majority of patients with FHI have only one eye affected, but the disease is bilateral in 7% to 15% of patients.

FHI is typically asymptomatic or presents with floaters or decrease in vision. It does not present with pain, redness, or photophobia.

FHI is an enigma because unlike most other forms of chronic anterior uveitis, patients with FHI do not develop posterior or anterior synechiae and, in the absence of surgery, do not develop cystoid macular edema (CME). This is the one form of anterior uveitis

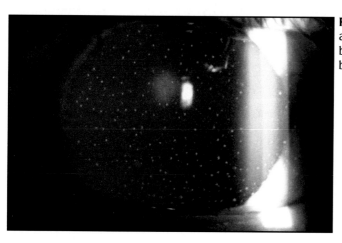

Figure 25-3. Stellate white KPs in a patient with FHI. Note the fibrin bridges, as well as the even distribution throughout the cornea.

that does not require aggressive therapy to completely quiet the anterior chamber. In fact, the inflammation of FHI rarely requires therapy. I have a few patients with FHI, however, who are so bothered by floaters resulting from anterior vitreous cells that I have offered periocular corticosteroid therapy, with the understanding that this treatment may not be beneficial and may hasten the development of cataract and, in steroid responders, increase the likelihood of glaucoma.

Patients with FHI are at increased risk of cataract, primarily posterior subcapsular cataract, and chronic glaucoma. The glaucoma is often resistant to medical therapy, requiring surgical management. Because the prevalence of glaucoma in FHI is at least 15%, intraocular pressure should be measured at least yearly and the optic nerve assessed for glaucomatous changes.

I manage the cataract in patients with FHI differently than other uveitic cataracts. Because the inflammation does not seem to cause damage and does not require therapy, the usual rule of 3 months of quiescence preoperatively does not apply. I used to pretreat FHI patients with corticosteroids, much as I do for other uveitic patients, but abandoned that practice years ago. I no longer treat FHI patients differently than routine (nonuveitic) cataract patients, with the exception that I discuss the increased risk of intraoperative or postoperative hyphema, secondary to the abnormal angle vessels associated with this condition. Patients who are very bothered by vitreous opacities may benefit from the addition of pars plana vitrectomy as well. The outcome of cataract and glaucoma surgery in FHI patients is usually excellent.[2,3]

Summary

Patients with FHI tend to present with inflammation that is asymptomatic. The inflammation may be discovered on routine examination or during an exam for floaters or decreased vision. The anterior chamber reaction responds minimally if at all to corticosteroid therapy and does not result in synechiae or CME. I tell patients with FHI that the prognosis for vision is generally excellent. I explain that the inflammation in this condition rarely requires therapy, and I counsel them about the need for regular follow-up because of the high incidence of glaucoma.

References

1. Rothova A, La Hey E, Baarsma GS, Breebaart AC. Iris nodules in Fuchs' heterochromic uveitis. *Am J Ophthalmol.* 1994;118:338-342.
2. Tejwani S, Murthy, Sangwan VS. Cataract extraction outcomes in patients with Fuchs heterochromic iridocyclitis. *J Cataract Refract Surg.* 2006;32:1678-1682.
3. La Hey E, de Vries J, Langerhorst CT, et al. Treatment and prognosis of secondary glaucoma in Fuchs' heterochromic iridocyclitis. *Am J Ophthalmol.* 1993;116:327-340.

How Do I Treat a Patient With Ocular Toxoplasmosis?

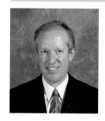

Gary N. Holland, MD

Toxoplasma gondii is the most common cause of retinal infections in otherwise healthy individuals, and it can cause severe, blinding disease in those with immunodeficiency states. Diagnosis is usually based on the typical appearance of a focal necrotizing lesion (Figure 26-1), often arising from the border of a pre-existing retinochoroidal scar, as recurrent disease (Figure 26-2). A substantial proportion of the general population is infected with *T. gondii*; therefore, serum antibody tests are usually of little diagnostic utility. I believe that it is appropriate to treat suspected lesions without laboratory confirmation (as might be obtained with PCR testing of vitreous humor specimens).

My choice of therapy for active disease depends primarily on the immune status of the patient. For the majority (those with normal host defenses), I treat with a combination of antimicrobial agents and corticosteroids, despite the fact that the value of such therapy has never been shown in well-designed clinical trials.[1] Most clinicians agree that treatment *does* have some beneficial effects, but lack of confirming evidence for any given treatment has resulted in a variety of drugs being used[2] (the fact that treatment efficacy has never been proven may simply reflect a lack of appropriate studies). By tradition, I still use "classic therapy" (pyrimethamine with folinic acid to reduce the risk of drug-associated side effects, sulfadiazine, and prednisone). Another, more convenient combination of a dihydrofolate reductase inhibitor and sulfonamide that is gaining increased popularity is trimethoprim/sulfamethoxazole (Bactrim, Septra). It is thought to be useful, despite animal studies showing it to be less effective than pyrimethamine/sulfadiazine. In patients who are allergic to sulfonamides, I use atovaquone as an alternative to pyrimethamine/sulfadiazine. Drug doses are listed in Table 26-1. With severe disease, I have occasionally added a fourth drug (clindamycin, the combination known as "quadruple therapy"[2]), although I am not convinced that it is more effective to do so.

Figure 26-1. A large retinochoroidal lesion in the left macula of an
immunocompetent adult with post-
natally acquired *Toxoplasma gondii*
infection. (Reprinted with permission of Holland GN. Ocular toxoplasmosis: a global reassessment.
Part II: disease manifestations and
management. *Am J Ophthalmol.*
2004;137:1-17, with permission
from Elsevier.)

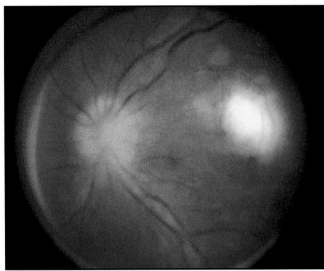

Figure 26-2. Recurrent toxoplasmic retinochoroiditis in an immunocompetent adult patient. There
is a "satellite lesion" associated
with pre-existing retinochoroidal
scars and a mild overlying vitreous
inflammatory reaction. (Reprinted
with permission of Holland GN.
Ocular toxoplasmosis: a global
reassessment. Part II: disease manifestations and management. *Am
J Ophthalmol.* 2004;137:1-17, with
permission from Elsevier.)

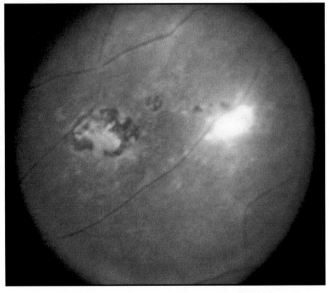

Table 26-1

Summary of Drug Therapy for Toxoplasmic Retinochoroiditis

Population	Drug	Dose	Duration	Comments
Immunocompetent individuals with active retinal lesions	Pyrimethamine	25 mg PO twice daily*	Until oral corticosteroid treatment is discontinued	
	Sulfadiazine	1 g PO qid	Same as above	
	Folinic acid	5 mg PO every other day	Until pyrimethamine is discontinued	
	Prednisone	40 to 60 mg PO daily (usually in divided doses)	Until vitreous inflammatory reaction decreases and retinal lesion borders harden	Begin 24 hours after start of antimicrobial agents
	Prednisolone acetate 1%	1 drop, 4 times daily	Until level of reaction is <1+ cells or resolution of redness and discomfort	Used if eye is red and uncomfortable or reaction is severe; anterior chamber cellular reactions will resolve without local treatment
Immunocompetent individuals with: (1) Inactive retinochoroidal scars adjacent to the fovea (2) Good visual acuity (3) A recent episode of active disease	TMP/SMX	One "double strength" tablet (TMP:160mg/ SMX: 800mg) PO every 3 days	2 years or longer	Treatment given as secondary prophylaxis to reduce risk of recurrence

(continued)

Table 26-1 (continued)

Summary of Drug Therapy for Toxoplasmic Retinochoroiditis

Population	Drug	Dose	Duration	Comments
Immunodeficient individuals	Pyrimethamine	25 mg PO twice daily*	Until lesion borders harden, at which time, one-agent maintenance therapy† is continued, as long as immunodeficiency state persists	Corticosteroids are not given
	Sulfadiazine	1 g PO qid	Same as above	
	Folinic acid	5 mg PO every other day	Until pyrimethamine is discontinued	
Individuals for whom pyrimethamine or sulfadiazine or both are not available or convenient	TMP/SMX	One "double strength" tablet (TMP: 160 mg/ SMX: 800 mg) PO twice daily (for treatment of active disease)	As per indications above	
Individuals with sulfonamide allergies	Atovaquone	750 mg PO twice daily (for treatment of active disease; once daily for secondary prophylaxis)	As per indications above	

TMP/SMX indicates trimethoprim/sulfamethoxazole; PO, by mouth; qid, four times daily.
*Loading dose (eg, 50 mg PO, given twice on the first day) may be administered, although clinical benefit has not been confirmed.
†TMP-SMX or atovaquone

I suspect that corticosteroids are the most important component of treatment for recurrent lesions in most otherwise healthy patients. It is likely that parasites reproduce for only brief periods of time and may already be encysted again in an inactive form by the time antimicrobials are taken. Corticosteroids limit the damaging effect of inflammation, but corticosteroids alone can lead to exacerbation of infection if active parasites are still present; antimicrobials protect against such proliferation. I wrote about many of these concepts in a comprehensive review, published elsewhere.[3]

Patients often have an anterior chamber cellular reaction, with redness and elevated intraocular pressure, at the onset of an active retinal lesion. Also by tradition, I treat those cases with a topical corticosteroid, but the risk of complications (eg, posterior synechiae) is small, and these reactions seem to resolve with systemic treatment alone. Elevated intraocular pressure will resolve without glaucoma medications.

With regard to duration of treatment, I continue drug therapy until lesion borders begin to "harden" and become more distinct (generally by 4 to 6 weeks), at which time I will rapidly taper and discontinue corticosteroids. I stop antimicrobials completely after corticosteroids have been stopped (antimicrobials should never be "tapered"). Vitreous haze may persist for months, but I do not consider it alone as an indication for continued treatment.

The goal of treatment is to hasten resolution, but because disease is self-limited with normal immune defenses, it is probably appropriate to observe some lesions without treatment, especially if they are small, in the peripheral retina, and without substantial vitreous haze. In that situation, I generally discuss the option of observation with patients, letting them decide whether to start treatment based on its potential risks, benefits, and expense. Patients who are observed without treatment should be followed closely; I reconsider treatment if vitreous haze increases and vision changes. Observation is an appropriate strategy for pregnant women with recurrent disease (a situation in which there is little potential for fetal damage because of pre-existing maternal antibodies). For pregnant women with newly acquired *T. gondii* infection, or with retinal lesions that are vision-threatening, choice of drug therapies should be made in conjunction with the patient's obstetrician and an infectious disease specialist.[2]

There is less doubt about the need for treatment of toxoplasmic retinochoroiditis in immunodeficient patients (eg, people with AIDS or those on immunosuppressive drug therapy). Without treatment, lesions will continue to enlarge, suggesting persistent parasite activity. Disease in elderly individuals may behave in a similar manner, probably because of waning host defenses. In such cases, I treat with antimicrobials alone. With persistent immunodeficiency, chronic therapy may be necessary. Options include trimethoprim/sulfamethoxazole or atovaquone; usually, one drug is sufficient.

In selected immunocompetent patients, I also administer long-term treatment as secondary prophylaxis to prevent recurrences. I do so based on a study undertaken in Brazil, in which trimethoprim/sulfamethoxazole, given every 3 days over a 20-month period, reduced the risk of recurrences.[4] I offer secondary prophylaxis to patients with histories of frequent recurrences or with lesions that would be immediately vision threatening with recurrence (eg, parafoveal lesions). If treatment is tolerated medically, I continue it for at least 2 years (when risk of recurrence is highest); however, some of my patients have elected to continue treatment for years. Regimens and alternatives were shown in Table 26-1.

References

1. Stanford MR, See SE, Jones LV, Gilbert RE. Antibiotics for toxoplasmic retinochoroiditis: an evidence-based systematic review. *Ophthalmology.* 2003;110:926-931.
2. Holland GN, Lewis KG. An update on current practices in the management of ocular toxoplasmosis. *Am J Ophthalmol.* 2002;134:102-114.
3. Holland GN. Ocular toxoplasmosis: a global reassessment. Part II: disease manifestations and management. *Am J Ophthalmol.* 2004;137:1-17.
4. Silveira C, Belfort R Jr, Muccioli C, et al. The effect of long-term intermittent trimethoprim/sulfamethoxazole treatment on recurrences of toxoplasmic retinochoroiditis. *Am J Ophthalmol.* 2002;134:41-46.

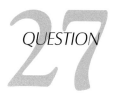

QUESTION

WHAT DISEASES SHOULD I CONSIDER
IN A PATIENT WITH NEURORETINITIS?

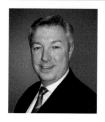

Emmett T. Cunningham, Jr, MD, PhD, MPH

Neuroretinitis is characterized by the triad of unilateral vision loss, optic disc edema, and macular star formation. It can occur at any age but most commonly affects children and young adults. Men and women are affected equally. Snellen visual acuity at presentation may vary from 20/20 to no light perception, and dyschromatopsia and an afferent papillary defect are common, although not always evident. Intraocular inflammation is typically nongranulomatous and mild. A peripapillary serous retinal detachment usually predates the formation of a macular star by 2 to 4 weeks. Once macular exudates do form, they tend to be most prominent in the papillomacular bundle, often producing an asymmetric or partial macular star (Figure 27-1). Systemic symptoms and signs are frequently absent, but should be elicited as some conditions known to cause neuroretinitis can be associated with prior or concurrent nonocular findings.

While the differential diagnosis list for neuroretinitis is long, up to two-thirds of cases in the developed world result from ocular *Bartonella henselae* infection. Most patients with *Bartonella*-associated neuroretinitis have a known exposure to cats or kittens, and many have a specific recollection of having been bitten or scratched. Supportive findings include a regional lymphadenopathy and the occurrence of focal retinitis or choroiditis. In addition to *B. henselae*, organisms known to cause neuroretinitis uncommonly include *Toxoplasma gondii*, *Treponema pallidum*, *Mycobacterium tuberculosis*, *Borrelia burgdorferi*, *Toxocara sp*, *Rickettsia typhi*, *Leptospira sp*, mumps virus, herpes viruses, and nematodes of the sort associated with diffuse unilateral subacute neuroretinitis (DUSN). Non-infectious etiologies include sarcoidosis and acute optic disc swelling in the setting of systemic vasculitis, such as Wegener disease, polyarteritis nodosa, and inflammatory bowel disease. Many cases of neuroretinitis remain idiopathic despite a thorough laboratory investigation.

Figure 27-1. Color photo montage of the right fundus of a patient with idiopathic neuroretinitis. The photograph was taken 5 weeks after the onset of symptoms and shows resolving optic disc edema with residual peripapillary subretinal fluid, a partial macular star, and retinal pigment epithelium mottling in and around the fovea. (Reprinted with permission of David Heiden, MD.)

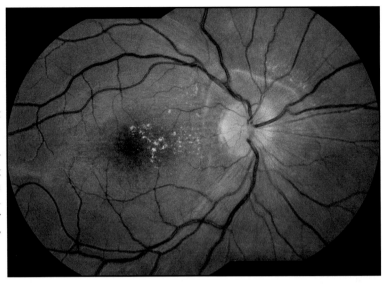

Bilateral neuroretinitis is rare and should prompt consideration of underlying conditions known to cause acute swelling of the optic disc, including malignant hypertension, diabetic papillitis, pseudotumor cerebri, and systemic vasculitis. Recurrent neuroretinitis is also uncommon but can occur, particularly in patients with ocular toxoplasmosis.

My diagnostic approach to the patient with neuroretinitis beyond history, review of systems, and eye examination is to first check blood pressure. Once malignant hypertension has been ruled out, I send the patient for fasting blood glucose, anti-*Bartonella* antibody titers, syphilis serology (including both an FTA-ABS and VDRL or RPR), a chest x-ray, an interferon-based TB test, and serum angiotensin-converting enzyme (ACE) and lysozyme levels. I typically also test for anti-*T. gondii* antibodies, particularly when there is a dense autoimmune progesterone dermatitis (APD), whitening of the peripapillary retina, or an adjacent or nearby retinochoroidal scar. I add Lyme testing when the patient lives in or has traveled to an endemic area and there is a known history of tick bite, erythema migrans, or arthritis. Leptospirosis is an important consideration in patients living or working in agricultural areas or with livestock, and is common in some developing world settings, but is generally uncommon in North America and Europe.

Most cases of neuroretinitis are either *Bartonella*-associated or idiopathic and, as such, typically resolve with or without treatment in 2 to 4 months. In fact, treatment of non-immunocompromised patients with neuroretinitis with systemic antibiotics has never been shown to be beneficial. That said, many choose to treat with systemic antibiotics, with options including doxycycline, ciprofloxacin, azithromycin, rifampin, intravenous gentamycin, and trimethoprim-sulfamethoxazole. I typically treat patients who present with neuroretinitis for presumed *Bartonella* infection with doxycycline 100 mg orally twice daily for 4 to 6 weeks. Erythromycin may be used in place of doxycycline in very young children where dental discoloration may be a concern. I modify this regimen if my initial laboratory workup supports a diagnosis other than *Bartonella* infection. Immunocompromised patients tend to need more aggressive treatment, including an extended 4-month regimen of doxycycline with or without rifampin, 300 mg orally twice daily. A short course of systemic corticosteroids, typically beginning with

0.5 mg/kg/day, may also be considered if the vision loss or intraocular inflammation is moderate to severe. Education and prevention are also important, including flea control and strict hand washing after handling cats or kittens.

The optic disc edema of neuroretinitis usually begins to resolve after 2 weeks and is typically fully resolved by 2 to 3 months. Macular exudates form approximately 2 to 4 weeks after the onset of symptoms and become increasingly apparent as the peripapillary fluid resorbs. Exudates begin to decrease after a month or so, but may take up to a year to resolve fully. Patients with heavy exudates may develop permanent alterations of the retinal pigment epithelium (see Figure 27-1), and some patients can be left with peripapillary gliosis and/or optic disc atrophy. While visual acuity returns to normal in all but the most severely affected patients, many continue to experience some sense of compromised vision. Recurrent disease is rare and has been suggested to be associated with a poorer visual prognosis. Toxoplasmic neuroretinitis, in particular, is recognized to be more likely to produce permanent changes in the patient's visual field and acuity.

Suggested Readings

Chappell MC, Jumper JM, McDonald HR, Cunningham ET Jr. Spotting *bartonella*-associated uveitis. *Review of Ophthalmology.* 2011;7:112-117.

Cunningham ET Jr, Koehler JE. Ocular bartonellosis. *Am J Ophthalmol.* 2000;130:340-349.

Ray S, Gragoudas E. Neuroretinitis. *Int Ophthalmol Clin.* 2001;41:83-102.

Roe RH, Michael Jumper J, Fu AD, Johnson RN, Richard McDonald H, Cunningham ET Jr. Ocular *Bartonella* infections. *Int Ophthalmol Clin.* 2008;18:93-105.

Suhler EB, Lauer AK, Rosenbaum JT. Prevalence of serologic evidence of cat scratch disease in patients with neuroretinitis. *Ophthalmology.* 2000;107:871-876.

WHAT ARE MY OPTIONS IN TREATING SYPHILITIC UVEITIS IN A PENICILLIN-ALLERGIC PATIENT?

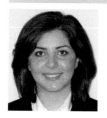

Lama Mulki, MD

Syphilis is a systemic disease caused by an infection by a spirochete known as *Treponema pallidum*, a thin, tightly wound, relatively stiff, spiral-shaped parasite measuring 10 to 13 μm. The disease may be classified as congenital or acquired. Congenital syphilis is usually diagnosed within the first 2 years of life, clinically or via the presence of immunoglobulin M (IgM) antibodies in the infant's blood. Acquired syphilis is sexually transmitted and should prompt the clinician to evaluate for other sexually transmitted diseases such as human immunodeficiency virus (HIV). It is usually divided into 3 different stages: primary syphilis with the hallmark being a chancre at the site of infection, secondary presented by generalized maculopapular rash as well as lymphadenopathy, and tertiary, which is usually characterized by gummatous lesions (granulomas) and involvement of the cardiovascular and central nervous system.

There has been a recent steady increase in the United States in the number of reported cases of primary and secondary syphilis since 2000, mostly among men. In 2007, the rate of primary and secondary syphilis is reported to be 3.8 per 100 000 population with an increase of 15.2% compared to 2006.[1] Diagnosis is made upon high level of clinical suspicion; treatment is usually curative.

What Are the Syphilitic Manifestations in the Eye?

Ocular syphilis can accompany any stage of the disease. It can involve any part of the eye and manifest like any other ocular inflammatory condition, thus the expression "the great masquerader." Examples include scleritis (which can be nodular or diffuse) and interstitial keratitis (which was the result of congenital syphilis in 90% of the cases prior to the antibiotic era or 1940s). Uveitis is the most common ocular manifestation, with syphilis being second only to tuberculosis as a cause of all uveitis cases prior to the 1940s. It can be granulomatous or nongranulomatous, can involve the anterior or the posterior part of the eye or both, and can be unilateral or bilateral. Patients may complain initially of nonspecific symptoms, such as photophobia, eye redness, and blurry vision. Findings may include iris nodules, roseolae of the iris, posterior synechiae, or lens dislocation. Syphilis can also manifest as chorioretinitis with grayish-yellowish-colored lesions involving the posterior pole or midperiphery. Retinitis without choroidal involvement may occur with intraretinal lesions seen on the fluorescein angiogram. Isolated retinal vasculitis, which can affect both arteries and veins, may also occur.[2-4]

How Is Ocular Syphilis Diagnosed?

Syphilis workup is usually the first step in the evaluation of any unexplained ocular inflammation, given the fact that it can mimic any other ocular inflammatory condition. The diagnosis is usually made by detailed history as well as serologies for both treponemal tests (FTA-ABS) and nontreponemal tests (VDRL-RPR). FTA-ABS should always be obtained in a patient with suspicious syphilis, because VDRL-RPR is only 70% sensitive in cases with primary or latent untreated syphilis. Darkfield examinations and direct fluorescent antibody (DFA) tests of a lesion exudate or the tissue remain the definitive methods for diagnosis. The practicing ophthalmologist should keep in mind that all patients with ocular syphilis should be evaluated for neurosyphilis with central spinal fluid analysis.

How Is Syphilitic Uveitis Usually Treated?

Treatment is as for neurosyphilis and consists of aqueous crystalline penicillin G 18 to 24 million units per day, administered as 3 to 4 million units intravenously every 4 hours or continuous infusion, for 10 to 14 days. If compliance with the therapy is an issue, the patient can be treated with Procaine penicillin 2.4 million units intramuscularly once daily, together with Probenecid 500 mg orally 4 times a day for 10 to 14 days.

Are There Any Alternatives for a Patient With Penicillin Allergy?

Parenteral penicillin remains the drug of choice for treatment of all stages of syphilis. This becomes problematic in a patient with penicillin allergy. The Centers for Disease Control and Prevention guidelines from 2006 recommend using penicillin whenever possible, especially in an HIV-positive patient.[5,6] Pregnant women with syphilis should be treated with penicillin as well. Therefore, penicillin skin allergy testing should be performed, provided the full battery of skin-test reagents is available. Patients who test negative can receive conventional penicillin therapy, while those who test positive should be desensitized. Alternatively, ceftriaxone can be used, although the possibility of cross-reactivity with penicillin exists. Ceftriaxone is usually used as 2 g daily either intramuscularly or intravenously for 10 to 14 days.

Other antibiotics as alternative regimens have not been studied sufficiently, and their routine use is not recommended. If patients are allergic to penicillin, either tetracycline or doxycycline may be considered. A penicillin-allergic patient with primary, secondary, or early latent syphilis who is HIV negative can be alternatively treated with doxycycline 100 mg orally twice daily or tetracycline 500 mg orally 4 times daily for 2 weeks, while late latent or tertiary syphilis and no evidence of neurosyphilis can be treated with doxycycline 100 mg orally twice daily or tetracycline 400 mg orally 4 times daily for 4 weeks.

As with any uveitis patient, topical, periocular, and systemic corticosteroids (orally or intravenously) also have an adjunctive role in the acute management of active inflammation. Ultimately, however, only timely administration of antibiotics renders a cure.

References

1. Centers for Disease Control and Prevention. *Syphilis surveillance report*. Centers for Disease Control and Prevention Web site. Retrieved from www.cdc.gov/std/Syphilis2007.
2. Kiss S, Damico FM, Young LH. Ocular manifestations and treatment of syphilis. *Semin Ophthalmol*. 2005;20:161-167.
3. Roque MR, Roque BL, Foster CS. *Ocular manifestations of syphilis*. Medscape Web site. Retrieved from http://emedicine.medscape.com/article/1202799-overview. Updated February 19, 2010.
4. Aldave AJ, King JA, Cunningham ET Jr. Ocular syphilis. *Curr Opin Ophthalmol*. 2001;12:433-441.
5. Centers for Disease Control and Prevention. Update to CDC's sexually transmitted diseases treatment guidelines, 2006: fluoroquinolones no longer recommended for treatment of gonococcal infections. *MMWR Morb Mortal Wkly Rep*. 2007;56:332-336.
6. Browning DJ. Posterior segment manifestations of active ocular syphilis, their response to a neurosyphilis regimen of penicillin therapy, and the influence of human immunodeficiency virus status on response. *Ophthalmology*. 2000;107:2015-2023.

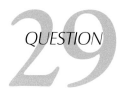

HOW DO I TREAT A PREGNANT WOMAN WITH A MACULA-THREATENING TOXOPLASMOSIS LESION?

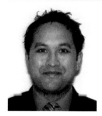

Rajiv Shah, MD

Toxoplasma gondii is the leading cause of infectious posterior uveitis worldwide. Macula- or vision-threatening retinochoroiditis or optic nerve involvement represents indication for treatment. However, unique to pregnancy is the urgency of preserving a mother's vision in addition to limiting, if not preventing, vertical transmission of the parasite, which may lead to severe comorbid effects or even termination of the pregnancy. Reactivation of congenital lesions is the classic teaching as to the etiology behind retinochoroiditis, but as more cases of acquired toxoplasmosis are recognized, this notion may change. Acquired toxoplasmosis commonly occurs from the consumption and handling of raw or undercooked meat (especially pork) or from the cleaning of cat litter boxes by pregnant women.

The approach to treatment in a pregnant patient is often intimidating because concerns arise with respect to which medication is safe for the fetus. Unfortunately, randomized controlled trials are simply not present for all classes of medications with respect to treating ocular toxoplasmosis. The standard scheme for summarizing the clinical evidence with respect to safety in pregnancy is as follow: "A" for safe as shown in human trials, "B" for presumed safe based on animal models, "C" for uncertain safety based on no human or animal trials, "D" for unsafe based on animal models, and "X" unsafe based on human trials. Currently, the only agents that carry a "D" rating are the tetracycline class. Thus, for pregnant woman and children, this class should not be considered unless all other options are exhausted or after an extensive risk/benefit discussion has been conducted with the patient and/or family. There are no known medications that are the "X" distinction. The only "A"-rated medication is folinic acid, which is used as an adjuvant to limit bone marrow toxicity when pyrimethamine therapy is used. The "B" category (macrolides, clindamycin, and atovoquone) or the "C" category (pyrimethamine/sulfadizine, Bactrim, and prednisone) will be discussed in more detail.

The macrolide class, in particular spiramycin, has the most human trial experience for the treatment of toxoplasmosis in pregnancy. Spiramycin is used 1 g every 8 hours for a period of 3 weeks. It has been a longstanding belief since the work of Desmonts and Couvreur that spiramycin decreased the rate of transmission by 60%. Recent multicenter European trials have challenged the notion that spiramycin prevents maternal fetal transmission, and recent work suggests that spiramycin does not cross the placenta to treat an infected fetus. This medication is not commercially available in the United States, but it can be obtained at no cost from Sanofi-Aventis after consultation with Food and Drug Administration (FDA), National Collaborative Treatment Trial Study, or Palo Alto Medical Foundation Toxoplasma Serology Laboratory. Azithromycin has not been as well studied in the setting of pregnancy, but there are limited data validating its safety. Azithromycin is used 500 mg daily. As will be discussed, pyrimethamine/sulfadiazine/folinic acid is considered the gold standard for treatment in the nonpregnant woman. A study evaluated the combination of pyrimethamine and azithromycin against the gold standard and found the end result to be equivalent between the 2 treatments with the notable exception that the azithromycin regimen was better tolerated. There is not enough evidence for azithromycin as monotherapy for the treatment of ocular toxoplasmosis.

The most classic treatment for toxoplasmosis centers on inhibition of the folic acid metabolism pathway of the parasite. Given the importance of folic acid metabolism for fetal neurologic development, this class of agents is contraindicated for usage in the first trimester. Pyrimethamine is the most effective anti-*Toxoplasma* agent. Pyrimethamine is given as a 100-mg loading dose with 25 to 50 mg daily for 30 to 60 days. It is coupled with sulfadiazine 1 g 4 times daily for synergistic antagonism of the folate acid metabolic pathway. Folinic 5 to 20 mg daily must be given with pyrimethamine to prevent bone marrow toxicity. Pyrimethamine/sulfadiazine/folinic acid is known as triple therapy and is considered the gold standard for treating *Toxoplasma*. One study compared it to other regimens (triple versus clindamycin versus Bactrim) and found that visual loss and recurrence rates were not different between regimens. The true benefit of triple therapy was that 49% of patients on triple therapy achieved smaller retinal lesion size and subsequently smaller retinal scars. Intolerance to medication, particularly to pyrimethamine, is the most common difficulty encountered with triple therapy. Bactrim DS, 1 tablet twice daily, inhibits folic acid in a similar fashion to triple therapy but is less toxic to the bone marrow and is better tolerated. Although clinical experience is more limited compared to triple therapy, a recent trial of Bactrim versus triple therapy demonstrated no difference in visual outcomes and/or retinal lesion size, contrary to the early comparison study.

Clindamycin used 300 mg 4 times a day for 30 to 40 days is another option. It has been coupled with the pyrimethamine/sulfadiazine/folinic acid as quadruple therapy. From animal models, clindamycin may reduce the number of Toxoplasma cysts, and it has been found to concentrate at the level of the retinal pigment epithelium, which is why lower doses are sufficient for treatment of retinochoroiditis. Furthermore, as a treatment for an obligate intracellular parasite such as toxoplasmosis, clindamycin has the advantage of increased intracellular concentration of nearly 3 times when compared to erythromycin.

Pseudomembranous colitis remains the dreaded complication of systemic clindamycin therapy, which occurs approximately 1/50,000 or 1/100,000 cases. Because chronic diarrhea may follow with many systemic antibiotic regimens, the recognition of pseudomembranous colitis requires vigilance and constant surveillance on the part of the practitioner. Despite these concerns with systemic usage, I am a strong supporter of this medication especially when used intravitreally for macula-threatening toxoplasmosis in pregnancy or otherwise. Clindamycin given intravitreally 1.0 mg/0.1 cc can be obtained locally or nationally through compounding pharmacies (such as Leiters). Intravitreal clindamycin has been shown to be highly effective as monotherapy in cases of medication intolerance in nonpregnant patients. The side effects and systemic delivery (and risk to the fetus) from intraocular injection are negligible if any. The typical dose has been found to be nontoxic to the retina with a half-life of 40 hours, sustaining levels above the 50% inhibitory concentration for toxoplasmosis. Some have advocated the co-injection with dexamethasone 400 mcg concomitantly with intravitreal clindamycin. A recent masked prospective trial evaluated intravitreal clindamycin with dexamethasone versus classic triple therapy with oral corticosteroids; the results demonstrated no difference in visual outcome and lesion size between the 2 regimens. Interestingly, there was a subgroup analysis that suggested that acquired toxoplasmosis, as indentified by positive immunoglobulin M (IgM) titers, may have reduced lesion size with systemic rather than intravitreal therapy. Although there is certainly a theoretical concern of creating a toxoplasmosis acute retinal necrosis with use of intravitreal corticosteroids, this trial and previous reports have not demonstrated this when antibiotics and steroids are injected together. As with any procedure, the risk of endophthalmitis, hemorrhage, damage to the crystalline lens, etc, must be discussed with the patient, but with proper technique and needles 30-ga or smaller, I find the benefits to outweigh the risks.

Atovoquone, an anti-malarial agent, is another option that may be better tolerated than the sulfa-based therapies. It is typically dosed 750 mg 4 times daily for 4 to 6 weeks. Although the experience for treatment of toxoplasma is also limited, this agent is widely used in treating malaria, especially in pregnancy with no known adverse effects to the fetus. There is a suspension form that increases the bioavailability, and in animal models, there has been a suggestion that Atovoquone may have activity against the cyst forms, which is poorly targeted by the more widely used agents for toxoplasma.

Corticosteroids are an adjunct to consider in addition to antimicrobial therapy. In retinochoroiditis, the use of steroids is thought to reduce the damage from the inflammation caused by toxoplasma. During pregnancy, the prolonged use of steroids may cause increases in cleft lips or palate, in addition to exacerbation of pregnancy-induced hypertension, gestational diabetes, osteoporosis, and infection. Close follow-up with a patient's obstetrician is necessary when systemic steroids are considered. One could consider periocular or intraocular steroids if the risks to the fetus are deemed unacceptable.

An additional consideration that bears mention in the pregnant patient revolves around maternal-fetal transmission. Recent longitudinal studies from Europe demonstrate an increase in vertical transmission with gestational age. The peak risk of transmission of 72% occurs around 36 weeks. These findings underscore some important nuisances. First, in an ideal scenario, close screening for toxoplasmosis antibodies titers through most prenatal visits would aid in early detection of a reactivation of latent maternal disease or newly acquired toxoplasmosis. Such screening is not routine in the United States but is mandated in some other countries. If there is a high concern for transmission to the fetus after 18 weeks of age, amniotic fluid sampling can be performed (although consideration must be given to the risk that such procedures pose to the fetus) and sent for PCR analysis. In one study, the PCR analysis had a sensitivity of 64% and a positive predicative value of 100% (a positive test means infection in the fetus). Ultrasound evaluations are also valuable to detect the possible fetal abnormalities such as hydrocephalus, calcification, or hepatosplenomegaly, which would be suggestive of toxoplasmosis. Current recommendations advocate Spiramycin for maternal infections prior to 18 weeks of gestation with a switch to pyrimethamine, sulfadiazine, and folinic acid after 18 weeks. The latter should also be used in cases where fetal infection has been confirmed.

Summary

Although there is no clear gold standard approach to the treatment of sight-threatening toxoplasmosis retinochoroiditis in pregnancy, I will suggest the following recommendations. Given the evolving evidence, I recommend intravitreal clindamycin for vision-threatening disease. One could consider reinjection after 3 days if necessary. The addition of concomitant intravitreal steroid is a matter of debate, but from the data available, I feel comfortable recommending it. With respect to the issue of concern for the fetus, I would recommend the macrolide class as first-line therapy, and this should be started as soon as possible, especially in the first trimester to protect the fetus from the severe consequences of vertical transmission. Although the bulk of the experience would indicate that Spiramycin should be the agent of choice, it is reasonable to use azithromycin or clarithromycin instead. As the patient approaches the 18-week gestation mark, a careful discussion of risk and benefit should be made regarding the amniotic fluid sampling and/or the switch to classic triple therapy. Certainly, other agents (such as atovoquone or combinations of pyrimethamine/azithromycin or pyrimethamine/atovoquone) can be considered given intolerance to medication or resistance to treatment, but there are fewer data and experience to guide outcomes and risk.

Suggested Readings

Foulon W, Villena I, Stray-Pedersen B, et al. Treatment of toxoplasmosis during pregnancy: a multicenter study of impact on fetal transmission and children's sequelae at age 1 year. *Am J Obstet Gynecol.* 1999;180 (2 Pt 1):410-415.

Kump LI, Androudi SN, Foster CS. Ocular toxoplasmosis in pregnancy. *Clin Experiment Ophthalmol.* 2005;33: 455-460.

Montoya J, Remington J. Management of *Toxoplasma gondii* infection during pregnancy. *Clin Infect Dis.* 2008;47: 554-566.

Sobrin L, Kump LI, Foster CS. Intravitreal clindamycin for toxoplasmic retinochoroiditis. *Retina.* 2007;27: 952-957.

Soheilian M, Ramezani A, Azimzadeh A, et al. Randomized trial of intravitreal clindamycin and dexamethasone versus pyrimethamine, sulfadiazine, and prednisolone in treatment of ocular toxoplasmosis. *Ophthalmology.* 2011;118:134-141. Epub 2010 Aug 12.

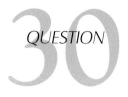

QUESTION

How Do You Treat Uveitis in Women Who Are Pregnant or Breastfeeding?

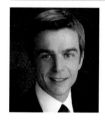

Erik Letko, MD

Noninfectious etiology and toxoplasmosis are, in my experience, the 2 most common causes of uveitis during pregnancy.

Noninfectious Uveitis

The rate of flare-ups of noninfectious uveitis during pregnancy is reported lower than during nonpregnant periods in the same group of women and lower than in the nonpregnant control group. Interestingly, the uveitis flare-ups tend to be more frequent in the first trimester and markedly less frequent in the second and third trimesters.[1,2] The reasons for decrease in likelihood of noninfectious uveitis flare-ups later in pregnancy remain poorly understood, but it is noteworthy that similar patterns of distribution of disease flare-ups during pregnancy and rebound postpartum were shown in patients with other autoimmune diseases, such as rheumatoid arthritis. Several hypotheses were postulated in the past to explain this phenomenon. These hypotheses include lack of adequate prevention of flare-ups with the use of immunomodulatory agents in order to avoid fetus- and newborn-related side effects during pregnancy and postpartum, respectively, and the presence of complex multifactorial intrinsic hormonal and cytokine changes that occur during this time period. The ones shown to play a role in maternal immunity include T helper cell types 1 and 2 cytokines, estrogen, alpha-2 pregnancy-associated globulin, maternal-fetal human leukocyte antigen incompatibility, and alpha-fetoprotein. As an example, increased production of maternal T helper cell type 1 proinflammatory cytokines during early pregnancy may account for an increase in the likelihood of flare-ups of noninfectious uveitis, while on the other hand, increased production of fetal-placental anti-inflammatory cytokines by

115

T helper cell type 2 and alpha-fetoprotein may account for decreased likelihood of flare-ups later in pregnancy. Similarly, an increase in secretion of proinflammatory cytokine prolactin may explain increased likelihood of flare-ups postpartum.

TREATMENT

I typically start treating a pregnant patient with an acute episode of noninfectious uveitis with an intensive topical regimen of corticosteroid drops such as difluprednate 0.05% or prednisolone acetate 1%. I ask the patient to press the lower lid punctum against the nose using the index finger for 5 minutes in order to reduce systemic absorption of the medication. Additionally, in patients with significant posterior segment inflammation, such as seen in Behçet's disease, Vogt-Koyanagi-Harada syndrome, or multifocal choroiditis, I administer periocular triamcinolone (40 mg/mL) via transseptal route. In cases with severe vision-threatening uveitis or when the inflammation does not respond well to topical or local corticosteroids, I will add, after consulting with patient's obstetrician, oral and/or intravenous corticosteroids. The dose of corticosteroids is tapered and discontinued over a period of 4 to 8 weeks, providing the patient and the fetus can tolerate the medication. For patients with noninfectious uveitis who continue to have significant inflammation that is vision-threatening despite the use of corticosteroids or while the corticosteroids are tapered or discontinued, one could consider implementing steroid-sparing immunomodulatory therapy with intravenous immunoglobulin after consultation with the patient's obstetrician.

Mydriatics and cycloplegic agents to prevent formation of posterior synechiae and to reduce discomfort from ciliary spasm should be used with caution during pregnancy due to potential side effects on the fetus. During pregnancy, I typically use homatropine 1% or 5% depending on severity of uveitis.

Ocular Toxoplasmosis

Ocular toxoplasmosis is, in my experience, the most common infectious uveitis encountered during pregnancy. Whether the association between pregnancy and ocular toxoplasmosis is causal remains unknown. Interestingly, according to one study, 4 of 7 women with an episode of toxoplasma uveitis had recurrence with each subsequent pregnancy.[3] According to another study, 3 of 4 pregnant women with toxoplasma uveitis ended up with permanent reduction in visual acuity despite aggressive therapy, suggesting that the course of disease might be more severe than that observed in nonpregnant women. The authors also noted that delivery may help recovery of toxoplasma uveitis in some patients.[4]

Ocular toxoplasmosis typically presents as a reactivation of an old chorioretinal lesion, which is a sign of congenital infection. In such a scenario, there is no transmission risk to the fetus. However, up to 20% of ocular toxoplasmosis cases might be acquired; therefore, it is important to consult with the patient's obstetrician and, when indicated, to pursue a full systemic work-up because the chance of transplacental infection is high. In case of acquired toxoplasmosis, the systemic treatment is driven by the obstetrician and/or infectious disease specialist.

TREATMENT

For pregnant women with ocular toxoplasmosis, I typically start treatment with an intensive regimen of corticosteroid drops such as difluprednate 0.05% or prednisolone acetate 1% along with an antibiotic regimen. The choice of antibiotic(s) depends on the stage of pregnancy, severity of inflammation, and proximity of the active chorioretinal lesion to the macula, optic disc, and/or major retinal vessels. I typically prescribe systemic antibiotics such as oral clindamycin (300 mg every 6 hours) with or without sulfadiazine (2 g loading dose followed by 1 g every 6 hours). Pyrimethamine (100 mg loading dose followed by 25 mg once a day) along with folinic acid (5 to 20 mg/day) could be added in severe cases where chorioretinal lesion threatens the macula, optic disc, or a major vessel. Azithromycin (500 to 1000 mg/day) could be used as an alternative. One has to keep in mind that pyrimethamine is contraindicated during the first trimester and sulfonamides are contraindicated in the third trimester. Some physicians prefer spiramycin (500 mg every 6 hours) as the drug of choice for ocular toxoplasmosis during pregnancy due to its decreased toxicity. However, spiramycin might be less effective compared to other alternative drugs, and in the United States it requires a special approval by the Food and Drug Administration. In cases with a significant amount of vitritis, I prescribe systemic corticosteroids starting at least 2 days after initiation of systemic antibiotics. I typically treat the patients with systemic antibiotics for 4 to 6 weeks. In cases where systemic therapy is contraindicated or where the clinical response to systemic therapy is not satisfactory, I use intravitreal clindamycin (1 mg/0.1 mL).[5,7] Alternatively, intraocular clindamycin can be used as first-line treatment in order to avoid potential teratogenic effects of systemic medications. The injection could be repeated in approximately 3 weeks. In case of severe vitritis, intraocular dexamethasone (0.4 mg/0.1 mL) can be used along with intravitreal clindamycin.[5,7] It is noteworthy that, in order to avoid undesirable drug-related side effects, patients with nonvision-threatening ocular toxoplasmosis can be observed without any antibiotic therapy.

Summary

Pregnancy in a patient with uveitis represents a therapeutic challenge. The treatment must be safe enough to avoid any teratogenic side effects, yet effective enough to halt inflammation and avoid vision loss of the pregnant woman. Accurate medical history, detailed eye exam, adequate counseling about the disease and prescribed medications, and frequent monitoring of response to treatment and side effects are critical when managing uveitis during pregnancy. A timely consultation with the patient's obstetrician and initiation of adequate therapy are keys to success.

References

1. Rabiah PK, Vitale AT. Noninfectious uveitis and pregnancy. *Am J Ophthalmol.* 2003;136:91-98.
2. Kump LI, Cervantes-Castaneda RA, Androudi SN, Foster CS, Christen WG. Patterns of exacerbations in chronic non-infectious uveitis in pregnancy and puerperium. *Ocul Immunol Inflamm.* 2006;14:99-104.

3. Bosch-Driessen LE, Berendschot TT, Ongkosuwito JV, Rothova A. Ocular toxoplasmosis: clinical features and prognosis of 154 patients. *Ophthalmology.* 2002;109:869-878.
4. Kump LI, Androudi SN, Foster CS. Ocular toxoplasmosis in pregnancy. *Clin Experiment Ophthalmol.* 2005;33: 455-460.
5. Martinez CE, Zhang D, Conway MD, Peyman GA. Successful management of ocular toxoplasmosis during pregnancy using combined intraocular clindamycin and dexamethasone with systemic sulfadiazine. *Int Ophthalmol.* 1998-1999;22:85-88.
6. Sobrin L, Kump LI, Foster CS. Intravitreal clindamycin for toxoplasmic retinochoroiditis. *Retina.* 2007;27: 952-957.
7. Lasave AF, Diaz-Llopis M, Muccioli C, Belfort R, Arevalo JF. Intravitreal clindamycin and dexamethasone for zone 1 toxoplasmic retinochoroiditis at twenty-four months. *Ophthalmology.* 2010;117:1831-1838.

HOW DO I DIAGNOSE AND TREAT ACUTE RETINAL NECROSIS?

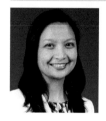

Suzanne Katrina V. Palafox, MD

Acute retinal necrosis (ARN) or Kirisawa-Urayama uveitis is part of a spectrum of necrotizing herpetic retinopathies.[1] Clinical evidence of ARN arises due to host and viral components. Our index of suspicion for ARN increases if this presents in a healthy individual. However, we should keep in mind that this condition is also seen in children and among immunocompromised individuals. ARN is reported to occur more frequently in males[2] peaking at ages 20 and 50 years.[3] Among White Americans, an association is seen between ARN and a HLA-DQβ0301 and phenotype Bw62, DR4,[4] while a Japanese study showed that some HLA antigens are statistically more common in the varicella-zoster virus (VZV)-ARN, but not in the herpes simplex virus (HSV) group.[5] VZV, HSV1 and 2, and cytomegalovirus (CMV) (infrequent) may all cause ARN.[1,2] VZV accounts for the majority; 14 of 17 ARN patients in a study established VZV as the etiologic agent.[6] ARN develops when the virus invades the retina intracellularly, which leads to retinal cell atrophy.[2,6] Pain, blurred vision, floaters, and constricted field of vision are key symptoms.[2] The American Uveitis Society's guidelines for diagnosing ARN include 1) retinal vaso-occlusion with arteriolar involvement, 2) sharply demarcated zones of necrotizing retinitis in peripheral retina, 3) circumferential spread, 4) rapid progression in the absence of antiviral therapy, 5) prominent vitritis, anterior chamber inflammation, 6) optic neuropathy[6] (Figure 31-1). Choroidal lymphocytic infiltrates and thickening are also helpful in confirming ARN. Performing a thorough anterior and posterior ophthalmologic examination is key, paying attention to the key features of ARN. We also keep in mind associated findings: retinal pigment epithelium (RPE) scarring anterior to the active border, retinal detachment, and recent or current meningitis or encephalitis.[2]

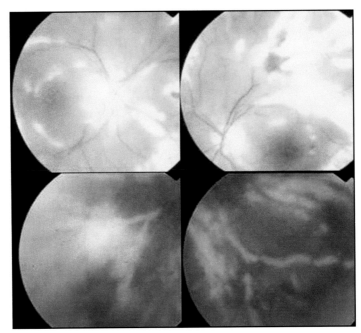

Figure 31-1. Dilated funduscopic exam revealed moderate vitritis, vasculitis, and extensive perivascular retinitis with areas of retinal hemorrhage and whitening.

Similar to any initial uveitis workup, an initial laboratory evaluation should include determining the presence of HSV 1 and 2, VZV, and CMV as possible causes of ARN; also determine the presence of VDRL and FTA-ABS, keeping in mind the differential diagnoses that can cause a necrotizing retinopathy picture. It is also prudent to investigate for antineutrophil cytoplasmic antibodies (ANCA) positivity, especially in cases where vasculitis may be the prominent feature to rule out systemic vasculitides. A pretreatment complete blood count (CBC) is warranted, as bone marrow suppression is a known adverse effect of antiviral agents, particularly for valganciclovir and ganciclovir. Obtaining a baseline blood urea nitrogen (BUN) and creatinine are also parameters to follow once therapy is commenced as some antiviral agents have nephrotoxic potential. Advice to the patients prior to starting treatment should include the potential of these agents to be carcinogenic and/or teratogenic.

Syphilitic neuroretinitis, acute multifocal hemorrhagic retinal vasculitis, CMV retinitis, Epstein-Barr virus (EBV) retinitis, toxoplasmic retinochoroiditis, *Candida albicans* endophthalmitis, Behçet's disease, sarcoidosis, progressive outer retinal necrosis (PORN), and primary intraocular lymphoma are all included in the realm of possible differential diagnoses.[1-3] We might be most confused in diagnosing ARN when faced with either of the first 2 entities mentioned.

In a recent study, polymerase chain reaction (PCR) studies detected the presence of genomic DNA for human herpes virus (HHV) in ocular fluids (68 aqueous humor and 43 vitreous fluid samples) of patients with uveitis. Among patients with ARN (n = 16), HSV1 was identified in 2 cases, HSV2 in 3 cases, while VZV was detected in 11 cases.[7]

Obtaining either aqueous or vitreous samples for PCR analysis is done to identify the etiologic agent.[1,7,8] It is controversial whether to pursue performing a vitreous tap, as this can be complicated by retinal detachment (2%)[1] or endophthalmitis. The Goldman-Witmer coefficient is useful too, more so in immunocompetent individuals, due to the high incidence of false negatives among immunocompromised individuals.[1]

The standard therapy for ARN is acyclovir given intravenously 10 mg/kg every 8 hours or 1500 mg/m[2] per day for 5 to 10 days, followed by oral acyclovir 800 mg 5 times daily for 6 weeks.[3] I agree with Tran and colleagues in maintaining the patient for a period of approximately 6 months to 1 year to cover for the period of high prevalence of bilateralization (4 months).[1] In another study, most patients received the following long-term antiviral treatment/prophylaxis under the newer antiviral era. These included valacyclovir 1000 mg daily to 1000 mg 3 times daily, famciclovir 250 to 500 mg twice daily, and valganciclovir 450 to 900 mg twice daily, aside from the more traditional oral acyclovir.[9] Anecdotal reports have demonstrated that valacyclovir 2000 mg 3 times daily has also been beneficial.

One may follow the recommendation of one study regarding the management of ARN, which entails prompt diagnosis; prophylactic argon laser retinopexy, preferably within the first 2 weeks to reduce risk of retinal detachment (RD); and systemic acyclovir, coupled with corticosteroids.[9]

Many experts believe that there is some value to performing a vitrectomy especially for dense vitreous opacities, including hemorrhage secondary to retinal neovascularization. Hillenkamp and colleagues described the benefit of using an early vitrectomy with intravitreal acyclovir lavage.[10] In this study, this approach was associated with a lower incidence of secondary RD; however, it did not improve mean visual acuity. Facilitating visualization to do prophylactic argon laser retinopexy is believed by a number of practitioners to be an important role for vitrectomy in managing ARN. Lau and colleagues reported rhegmatogenous retinal detachment (RRD) in 35.3% of eyes that received prophylactic laser treatment versus 80% in eyes that did not. It is recommended to perform laser treatment at least 2 weeks after onset of retinitis to prevent RD.[11]

We may choose to use methylprednisolone 500 mg/kg for 3 days and continue with oral prednisone (1 mg/kg/day) with a slow taper for 4 to 6 weeks. Heparin can be employed to help prevent occlusive vasculitis or acetylsalicylic acid (250 mg/day).[1]

The visual prognosis of ARN is poor, particularly in VZV-induced cases.[2,5]

I recommend adhering to the criteria for intensive treatment proposed for the diseases under the umbrella of necrotizing herpetic retinopathies to be applied to selected cases of ARN: 1) immunocompromised state, 2) bilateral ARN, 3) monocular patients, 4) extension of retinal involvement, threatening more than 2 quadrants and/or posterior pole, 5) antecedent resistance to acyclovir, and 6) absence of response to treatment after 2 days.[1] This treatment consists of intravenous foscarnet (60 mg/kg every 8 hours during 2 or 3 weeks, followed by a maintenance dosage of 90 mg/kg/day) plus intravitreal ganciclovir (200 to 2000 µg/0.1 mL).[1] Tibbetts and colleagues advocate intravitreal foscarnet (1.2 to 2.4 mg per 0.1 mL) or intravitreal ganciclovir (200 to 2000 µg/0.1 mL) as adjunctive therapy to oral antiviral agents.[9] ARN is a very complex disease with many possible entities that resemble it. If ophthalmologists are clear on remembering the key diagnostic features, coupled with the positive supporting parameters in the ancillary evaluation, one can then confidently diagnose this potentially blinding disease and provide the necessary treatment. Time is of the essence in identifying and treating ARN. The index of suspicion arises when we are faced with a patient with pain, blurred vision, floaters, and a constricted field. In performing a detailed exam, we must be careful to search for anterior segment hyperemia, iritis, vitreous inflammation, peripheral confluent retinal necrosis, satellite lesions, optic nerve edema/pallor, and retinal vascular occlusion. Associated findings may include RPE scarring anterior to the active border, serous RD or RRD, and a coinciding recent or current meningitis or encephalitis.[2]

References

1. Tran TH, Bodaghi B, Rozenberg F, Cassoux N, Fardeau C, LeHoang P. Viral cause and management of necrotizing herpetic retinopathies. *J Fr Ophthalmol.* 2004;27:223-236.
2. Davis JL, Fox GM, Blumenkranz MS. Acute retinal necrosis. In: Albert DM, Miller JW, Azar DT, Blodi BA. *Albert and Jakobiec's Principles and Practice of Ophthalmology.* 3rd ed. Ontario, Canada: Saunders Elsevier; 2008:2115.
3. Nussenblatt RB, Whitcup SM. *Uveitis: Fundamentals and Clinical Practice.* 3rd ed. Philadelphia, PA: Mosby; 2004:201-202.
4. Holland GN, Cornell PJ, Park MS, et al. An association between acute retinal necrosis syndrome and HLA-DQw7 and phenotype Bw62, DR4. *Am J Ophthalmol.* 1989;108:370-374.
5. Ichikawa T, Sakai J, Yamauchi Y, Minoda H, Usui M. A study of 44 patients with Kirisawa type uveitis. *Nippon Ganka Gakkai Zasshi.* 1997;101:243-247.
6. Holland GN. Standard diagnostic criteria for the acute retinal necrosis syndrome. Executive Committee of the American Uveitis Society. *Am J Ophthalmol.* 1994;117:663-667.
7. Sugita S, Shimizu N, Watanabe K, et al. Use of multiplex PCR and real-time PCR to detect human herpes virus genome in ocular fluids of patients with uveitis. *Br J Ophthalmol.* 2008;92:928-932.
8. Lau CH, Missotten T, Salzmann J, Lightman SL. Acute retina necrosis features, management, and outcomes. *Ophthalmology.* 2007;114:756-762.
9. Tibbetts MD, Shah CP, Young LH, Duker JS, Maguire JI, Morley MG. Treatment of acute retinal necrosis. *Ophthalmology.* 2010;117:818-824.
10. Hillenkamp J, Nölle B, Bruns C, Rautenberg P, Fickenscher H, Roider J. Acute retinal necrosis: clinical features, early vitrectomy and outcomes. *Ophthalmology.* 2009;116:1971-1975,e2.
11. Lau CH, Missotten T, Salzmann J, Lightman SL. Acute retinal necrosis: features, management and outcomes. *Ophthalmology.* 2007;114:756-762.

HOW DO I DIAGNOSE AND TREAT POSNER-SCHLOSSMAN SYNDROME?

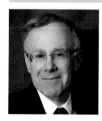

Howard H. Tessler, MD

The Posner-Schlossman syndrome (PSS; glaucomatocyclitic crisis) is uncommon and tends to be overdiagnosed by residents. It is a diagnosis of exclusion. Just because a patient presents with an elevated intraocular pressure and anterior uveitis does not establish the diagnosis as the PSS.

The symptoms of PSS are more like those of angle-closure glaucoma than acute anterior iritis. Patients complain of vague aching, halos, and blurred vision. They seldom have severe pain and photophobia. It is usually unilateral. PSS usually presents in the third to seventh decade of life.

On examination, there is no injection or only low-grade erythema of the conjunctiva. Frequently, the pupil is slightly dilated and not miotic as in other cases of acute iritis. Microcystic edema of the cornea can be present along with a few nongranulomatous keratic precipitates (KP; Figure 32-1). The anterior chamber has low-grade inflammation, such as 1 to 2+ flare and less than 2+ cells. Synechia do not form. The intraocular pressure (IOP) can be quite elevated. Frequently, the IOP reaches above 40 mm Hg, even to the 60s. It has been hypothesized that PSS is a trabeculitis. One case treated with a trabeculectomy during an acute attack was found to have numerous mononuclear cells in the trabeculum.[1]

These patients do not have posterior findings unless they develop glaucomatous cupping. They do not develop cystoid macular edema (CME). The typical attack lasts 4 days to 2 weeks. Patients may have multiple recurrences, and over time mild diffuse hypochromia of the involved iris may occur. The heterochromia in PSS is much less evident and pronounced than in Fuchs' heterochromic iridocyclitis (FHI; Figure 32-2).

Figure 32-1. Note small number of KP and epithelial edema of cornea.

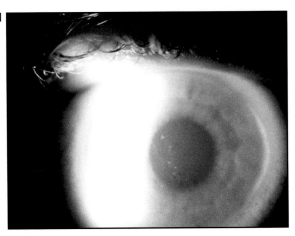

Figure 32-2. Left eye shows mild pupillary mydriasis and iris hypochromia in patient who has had multiple attacks of Posner Schlossman syndrome.

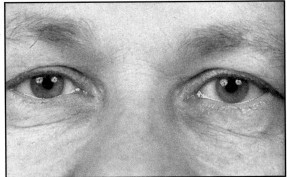

The differential diagnosis of PSS includes other causes of unilateral iritis and elevated IOP. Herpes simplex virus (HSV) and herpes zoster virus (VZV) iritis can be confused, especially if there is no evidence of corneal disease or a history of shingles. In herpetic uveitis, sectoral stromal atrophy, iris transillumination defects, and chronicity help make a separation from PSS. FHI is chronic, and the secondary glaucomatous elevation is usually not as dramatic as in PSS. Sarcoidosis should be considered as a cause of any uveitis; however, it usually causes a chronic inflammation, with granulomatous features and the formation of synechia (Table 32-1). Acute human leukocyte antigen (HLA)-B27 iritis is usually unilateral, but there is severe pain and photophobia with a miotic pupil, the tendency to form synechia, and severe inflammation.

The etiology of PSS is uncertain. A herpetic cause has been hypothesized, and a study from Boston in 1995 found aqueous humor polymerase chain reaction (PCR) evidence of HSV in 3 cases.[2] These cases were negative for cytomegalovirus (CMV) and VZV. In 2008, a study from Singapore reported that 37.5% of 18 patients with PSS had CMV positivity on aqueous PCR.[3] These patients had normal immunity. These eyes were negative for HSV and VZV. They also had 30 patients with PSS who were negative for all viruses. Thus, there seems to be an association with the herpes virus family in some cases. The etiology of this condition appears to be multifactorial.

Table 32-1
Differential Diagnosis of Posner-Schlossman Syndrome

Syndrome	Time	Pupil	Synechia	Iris
Posner-Schlossman syndrome	Acute, short duration	Pupil slightly dilated	No synechia	Late mild stromal atrophy
Fuchs' heterochromic iridocyclitis	Chronic	Pupil not affected	No synechia	Diffuse stromal atrophy
Herpes simplex virus and herpes zoster virus	Chronic	Pupil may be atonic and large	Can have synechia	Sectoral stromal and pigment epithelial atrophy
Sarcoid	Chronic	Miotic	Yes synechia	No atrophy
HLA-B27	Acute	Miotic	Yes synechia	No atrophy

The treatment of PSS is aimed at lowering the IOP. Patients can be treated with topical beta-blockers, topical or oral carbonic anhydrase inhibitors, and alpha agonists such as brimonidine. Whether topical prostaglandins should be used is uncertain. In my experience, if a topical corticosteroid is used, the prostaglandin drugs seem well tolerated and do not seem to increase inflammation.

Most uveitis specialists use topical corticosteroids in addition to antihypertensives. Corticosteroids such as rimexolone (Vexol), loteprednol (Lotemax), or fluorometholone (FML) should be considered instead of strong drugs such as 1% prednisolone or difluprednate (Durezol). Usually, the corticosteroids are used 4 times daily and then tapered as these attacks subside.

There is evidence that some of these patients develop sustained elevated IOP leading to chronic glaucoma after numerous attacks over the years.

Because of evidence of some herpetic viruses as a possible etiology, it is worth considering an anterior chamber tap and ordering PCR looking for HSV and CMV. The result of treatment for CMV in these cases is somewhat encouraging. Patients have been variably treated with IV and oral ganciclovir, oral valganciclovir, and intravitreal ganciclovir. Patients showed improvement with either no attacks or less severe and less frequent attacks, but 9 of 12 patients had recurrences on stopping therapy. Because PSS is so variable in recurrence (months to years), it is difficult to tell how successful therapy is. In my personal experience with oral valganciclovir therapy in 2 patients with positive aqueous PCR for CMV, treatment did not seem to stop recurrences.

References

1. Harstad HK, Rinvvold A. Glaucomatocyclitic crises (Posner-Schlossman syndrome). A case report. *Acta Ophthalmol.* 1986;64:146-151.

2. Yamamoto S, Pavan-Langston D, Tada R, et al. Possible role of herpes simplex virus in the origin of Posner-Schlossman syndrome. *Am J Ophthalmol.* 1995;119:796-798.
3. Chee S-P, Bacsal K, Jap A, et al. Clinical features of cytomegalovirus anterior uveitis in immunocompetent patients. *Am J Ophthalmol.* 2008;145:834-840.

WHAT IS IMMUNE RECOVERY UVEITIS AND HOW DO I TREAT IT?

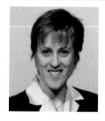

Jennifer E. Thorne, MD, PhD

Cytomegalovirus (CMV) retinitis, a common ocular opportunistic infection among patients with HIV/AIDS, was estimated to affect 30% of patients with AIDS prior to the introduction of highly active antiretroviral therapy (HAART). HAART-induced immune recovery (defined as an increase in CD4+ T cell count to 100 or more cells/μL) has resulted in a declining number of opportunistic infections, including an approximate 80% reduction in the incidence of CMV retinitis. Patients with CMV retinitis and immune recovery have a better prognosis with a lower risk of retinitis progression, retinitis-related retinal detachment, second eye involvement, visual acuity and visual field loss, and mortality.[1]

However, the benefits of HAART may be attenuated by the development of immune recovery uveitis (IRU), which is characterized by intraocular inflammation (commonly intermediate uveitis or a combination of anterior and intermediate uveitis), in conjunction with immune recovery, and may be associated with ocular complications such as cataract, cystoid macular edema (CME), and epiretinal membrane (ERM) formation. A proposed pathogenesis for IRU is that immunologic improvement in response to HAART causes the restoration of specific anti-CMV immunity, which leads to an inflammatory response directed at the CMV antigen present in the eye. Immune recovery uveitis may occur soon after initiating HAART (less than 1 month), but also has been reported to occur as long as 3 years after starting HAART. The prevalence of IRU has been estimated at 18% to 25% depending on the series, and the incidence of IRU in patients with CMV retinitis is estimated at 10% to 20% per year. Treatment of CMV retinitis with intravenous cidofovir and large CMV lesion size have been reported to increase the risk of IRU.[2,3] Patients with CMV retinitis who do not have HIV/AIDS also may develop IRU if their immune systems improve. For example, a patient who develops CMV retinitis while receiving immunosuppressive drug therapy for graft versus host disease may develop IRU as a consequence of having the immunosuppressive drug therapy discontinued.

The most common structural ocular complications of IRU are CME, ERM, and cataract. Other reported complications of IRU include optic disc edema, optic disc and retinal neovascularization, and neovascular glaucoma. IRU and its attendant complications may result in loss of visual acuity.[2-4] Typically, the visual acuity loss is mild to moderate (visual acuities worse than 20/40 but better than 20/200). Among eyes with CMV retinitis in patients with immune recovery, IRU and its complications (CME, cataract, and ERM) resulted in 45% to 50% of the incident loss of visual acuity in a large multicenter prospective cohort study.[4]

The treatment of IRU depends on the location of the intraocular inflammation, the severity of the inflammation, and the presence of ocular complications, particularly CME. Inflammation in the anterior chamber is treated with topical corticosteroids in frequencies typical of treating other forms of anterior uveitis, typically prednisolone acetate 1% drops dosed every 1 to 2 hours while awake for 2 to 4 weeks followed by a taper. If the IRU is an isolated mild vitritis without CME, these eyes may be observed, as the vitreous inflammation can be transient. Immune recovery uveitis with more severe vitreous inflammation and/or CME typically is treated with periocular corticosteroids (triamcinolone acetonide 40mg), or short courses of oral corticosteroids, without recurrence of the CMV retinitis. In unilateral IRU cases, I typically will treat with a periocular corticosteroid injection and re-evaluate the patient in 1 month to determine if additional injections are required. In cases of bilateral IRU or among patients with inadequate response to periocular injections, I will treat with oral prednisone, typically 1mg/kg/day (up to 60mg daily) for 2 to 4 weeks followed by a taper. I will supplement this therapy with topical nonsteroidal anti-inflammatory drugs for eyes with partial resolution of CME. The majority of patients treated will have a decrease in IRU-associated CME and improvement in visual acuity. Although treatment with valganciclovir has been reported to improve visual acuity among patients with IRU-related CME in small case series, I typically do not add valganciclovir to the treatment regimen.

References

1. Jabs DA, Bartlett JG. AIDS and ophthalmology: a period of transition. *Am J Ophthalmol.* 1997;124:227-233.
2. Zegans ME, Walton RC, Holland GN, et al. Transient vitreous inflammatory reactions associated with combination antiretroviral therapy in patients with AIDS and cytomegalovirus retinitis. *Am J Ophthalmol.* 1998;125:292-300.
3. Kempen JH, Min YI, Freeman WR, et al; Studies of Ocular Complications of AIDS Research Group. Risk of immune recovery uveitis with AIDS and cytomegalovirus retinitis. *Ophthalmology.* 2006;113:684-694.
4. Thorne JE, Jabs DA, Kempen, JH, Holbrook JT, Nichols C, Meinert CL; Studies of Ocular Complications of AIDS Research Group. Causes of visual acuity loss among patients with AIDS and CMV retinitis in the era of highly active antiretroviral therapy. *Ophthalmology.* 2006;113:1441-1445.

HOW DO I EVALUATE AND TREAT A PATIENT WITH RETINAL VASCULITIS?

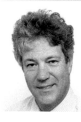

William Ayliffe, FRCS, PhD

Retinal vasculitis is a clinical term describing inflammatory disease of the retinal vasculature, seen as focal cuffing, segmental sheathing, hemorrhage, and local perivascular inflammatory response (Figure 34-1). Ischemia causes cotton-wool spots and neovascularization of the retina or optic nerve (Figure 34-2). Subtle signs may only be revealed by fluorescein angiography. Retinal vasculitis is not a single disease but a response to various insults. Some are restricted to the eyes, but others represent a manifestation of systemic disease or infection. The eye may be their herald organ. Some systemic diseases may not manifest for years after their initial presentation as retinal vasculitis.

A number of causes are possible, from idiopathic to ocular or systemic disease.

Infections (eg, toxoplasmosis, herpetic retinitis, tuberculosis, and syphilis) must be considered in certain high-risk groups. Systemic inflammatory diseases, such as sarcoidosis, multiple sclerosis, and Behçet's disease, may develop or even present with retinal vasculitis. Finally, some cases are caused by localized disease of the eye, such as pars planitis, birdshot retinochoroidopathy, Eale disease (in high-risk populations), and idiopathic retinal vasculitis.[1]

Retinal vasculitis typically presents with floaters and painless blurring of vision.

Clinical history may reveal occult or active systemic disease: cough and loss of weight occurs in sarcoid and chronic infection; rashes or Raynaud phenomenon in systemic vasculitis; mouth ulcers suggest Behçet's. With residence or travel to endemic locations, suspect Lyme disease or Rickettsial causes. Ask about risk factors for human immunodeficiency virus.

On examination, iritis may be minimal or severe with granulomatous keratic precipitates in viral retinitis, vasculitides, and sarcoidosis. Hypopyon develops in some patients with Behçet's disease. Patients with primary retinal vasculitis or birdshot

Figure 34-1. Fundus photograph showing nipping of the veins.

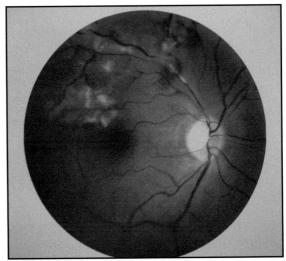

Figure 34-2. Fundus photograph disclosing creamy white cuffs of perivascular exudation of inflammatory cells.

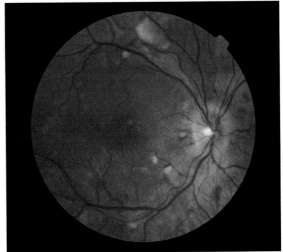

retinochoroidopathy may have minimal vitritis. A dense vitreal inflammation occurs in sarcoid but is highly suspicious of infective causes, particularly toxoplasmosis or herpetic retinal necrosis in immunocompetent individuals. Vitreous hemorrhage is a presenting feature of Eale disease. Periphlebitis is the hallmark of retinal vasculitis; initially, nipping of the veins is observed, and later, creamy white cuffs of perivascular exudation of inflammatory cells develop (see Figure 34-1). Inactive areas of old disease show grey fibrous sheathing of the vessels. Arteritis is less common.

Patches of retinal whitening due to focal retinal necrosis is seen in Behçet's, and pigmented borders suggest toxoplasmosis. More extensive peripheral necrosis occurs in herpetic retinitis.

Routine investigations should include chest x-ray, full blood count, sedimentation rate, and serology for syphilis and Lyme. human leukocyte antigen (HLA) typing and autoimmune screening are indicated by history. Anergy to Mantoux in patients who have had Bacillus Calmette-Guérin (BCG) immunization suggests sarcoidosis.

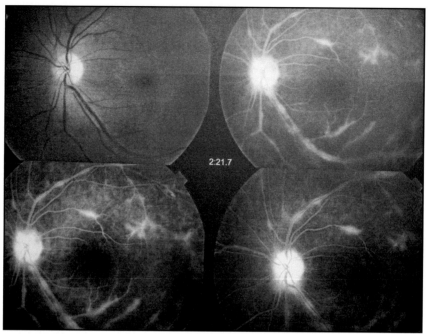

Figure 34-3. Fluorescein angiography showing papillitis, phlebitis and multifocal vasculitis.

Fluorescein angiography delineates the extent of the disease and reveals occult sites of inflammation and leakage. It also outlines the ischemic areas in occlusive vasculitis that can direct focal retinal laser treatment (Figure 34-3). Biopsy of vitreous, retina, lymph nodes, or even nerve may be indicated to exclude masquerading conditions.[2]

Treatment is not always necessary. When changes are mild, observation is sufficient. Sight-threatening lesions require systemic anti-inflammatory and, if appropriate, anti-infective medication. Topical therapy is used for iritis or glaucoma. The aim is to get rapid control to minimize damage. Once achieved, steroid-sparing immunomodulatory therapy (IMT) avoids the inevitable long-term side effects of prolonged steroid therapy. Once infection has been excluded or treated, high-dose prednisone (1 mg/kg/day, reduced by 10 mg/day each week if no relapse to 10 mg/day maintenance) is initiated. If disease is not controlled, IMT is introduced. Anti-metabolites, methotrexate, mycophenolate mofetil, and azathioprine have a slow onset but a low rate of serious side effects. If rapid control of disease is required, cyclosporine or tacrolimus is used. These expensive drugs require careful monitoring. In general, they are not used for very long-term control.[3]

Third-line therapy includes anti-tumor necrosis factor (TNF) antibodies, infliximab infusions, or Humira injections. For Behçet's, interferon therapy has a role. Alkylating drugs, typically cyclophosphamide, are occasionally used—particularly in cases of systemic vasculitis.

Retinal photocoagulation is required for obliterative vasculitides, Eale disease, cases of focal ischemia, and as an alternative to cryotherapy in some cases of pars planitis (Figure 34-4). Vitrectomy can be considered to clear persistent inflammatory debris or hemorrhage and to remove epiretinal membranes. Retinal tears and detachment, particularly cases of acute retinal necrosis, require vitreoretinal intervention.

Figure 34-4. Fundus photograph showing peripheral neovascularization along with sub-hyaloid hemorrhage.

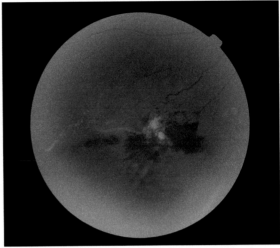

References

1. Nussenblat RB, Whitcup SM, Palestine AG. *Uveitis, Fundamentals and Clinical Practice.* 3rd ed. Philadelphia, PA: Mosby; 2004.
2. Foster CS, Vitale AT. *Diagnosis and Treatment of Uveitis.* Philadelphia, PA: WB Saunders; 2003.
3. Jabs DA, Rosenbaum JT, Foster CS, et al. Guidelines for the use of immunosuppressive drugs in patients with ocular inflammatory disorders: recommendations of an expert panel. *Am J Ophthalmol.* 2000;130:492-513.

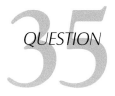

How Do I Approach a Patient With Exudative Retinal Detachment and Uveitis?

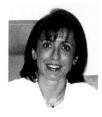

Margarita Calonge, MD

An exudative retinal detachment (RD) can occur as a consequence of severe inflammation in the choroid with resultant retinal pigment epithelium (RPE) damage, producing a secondary breakdown of the external blood-retina barrier. This breakdown will accumulate subretinal fluid, forming localized areas of serous RD or, if more intense, total exudative RD with bullous appearance.

It is crucial to distinguish exudative RD from rhegmatogenous RD, traction RD, retinoschisis, and choroidal effusions. A rhegmatogenous RD must always be carefully ruled out because the therapeutic approach in this case is always surgical. To be absolutely sure about this possibility, retinal periphery has to be examined for a retinal hole or tear. To this aim, I usually have these patients examined initially by a retinal specialist before proceeding with medical treatment for exudative RD.

Exudative RD can be associated with several types of uveitis, but it is more characteristic of specific conditions such as Vogt-Koyanagi-Harada (VKH) disease, whose ocular hallmarks involve severe bilateral panuveitis associated with exudative RD. Again, differential diagnosis with rhegmatogenous RD is crucial, as the latter can also occur in VKH. Nonrhegmatogenous RDs in VKH are usually seen as early manifestations of the disease in the acute stage[1] and do not usually persist after initial presentation, and one can later see demarcation lines representing the extent of previous RD. Large choroidal granulomas, can be seen in sarcoidosis (yellow-white or yellow-gray discrete elevated masses can have overlying serous RD). Other diseases can actually have serous RD among their findings, such as infectious uveitis due to bartonella henselae (cat-scratch disease), borreliosis (Lyme disease), rickettsia conorii (Mediterranean spotted fever), tuberculosis, or syphilis. Choroidopathy in association with systemic lupus erythematosus has been reported in conjunction with serous elevations of the RPE and sensory retina, some progressing to large, bullous, exudative RD, which resolved after control of the disease. A serous exudative RD has been described as characteristic of hypotony maculopathy. Masquerade syndromes such as lymphoma, leukemia, or melanoma can also manifest with exudative RD. Finally, it is also known that certain drugs can cause serous RD, such as systemic corticosteroids or interferon therapy.

Management

Exudative RD is the manifestation of choroidal inflammation, RPE dysfunction, and therefore retinal barrier breakdown. Management is always through medical therapy and it is aimed at controlling inflammation. With aggressive therapy, one can assume that nonrhegmatogenous RD will reattach. This reattachment usually results in reasonably good vision, although permanent changes can actually preclude regaining previous visual acuity (RPE stippling, pre-retinal membranes, subtle folds in the retina, posterior pole atrophy, or even subretinal fibrosis).

If the serous RD occurs in the context of an infectious problem, it is my experience that specific anti-infective treatment will resolve inflammation, and therefore, once the RPE starts functioning again, the subretinal fluid will be reabsorbed.

In the most frequent case of exudative RD, which is in the context of VKH disease, aggressive therapy is started with corticosteroids as the drug of choice. They are usually given systemically, starting at a dose of 1 mg/kg/day. In cases of more severe inflammation, bilateral RD and a substantial drop in visual acuity starting dose can be 2 mg/kg/day or even intravenous high-dose pulse steroids, usually 1000 mg/day of methylprednisolone for 3 consecutive days, followed by 1 mg/kg/day orally. In the 2 latter circumstances, it is wise to hospitalize patients for a careful follow-up and prevention of potential complications. There is controversy as to whether to start with intravenous pulse steroids, as it has been reported not to be better than the oral route.[2] I usually begin with 1.5 mg/kg/day, with no hospitalization but close follow-up (involving family doctors) and always add a second immunosuppressant as a first-line therapy from the beginning (usually cyclosporine) as this regimen seems to be superior to steroids as monotherapy or delayed addition of immunotherapy.[3]

Intravitreal corticosteroids for this condition were not usually recommended in the past, as injections can be problematic, particularly in large detachments. In particular cases in which high doses of systemic steroids cannot be given and provided the RD is not very large, I have used one single injection of intravitreal triamcinolone, usually followed by moderate doses of steroids and cyclosporine if possible. Recently, a refractory case of exudative RD due to VKH syndrome was treated with an intravitreal injection of bevacizumab with a spectacular fast recovery of the multiple serous RD.[4] Repeated injections, however, must be avoided, as they may create a hole, compounding the problem. In this regard, the use of fluocinolone acetonide implants (Retisert) has been documented in 2 patients with VKH and serous RD as of limited use, as corticosteroids could not be fully tapered off.[5] Finally, intravitreal dexamethasone implants, which have become commercially available recently, could be indicated in this type of RD, although there are not yet published experiences.

Before intravitreal anti-vascular endothelial growth factor (VEGF) therapy was available, we reattached the retina of 2 VKH patients where correct medical therapy had failed in the fellow eye. When the second eye got involved, and after failure of high-dose steroid therapy plus cyclosporine, patients underwent vitrectomy plus injection of intraocular silicone (which was removed after 3 months) as the subretinal fluid will not be reabsorbed by a diseased RPE. Both cases were successfully reattached, and vision was regained in the only remaining eye. No retinal tear was ever found.

Summary

An accurate diagnosis of exudative RD versus mainly rhegmatogenous RD must be made first, followed by great efforts to find the etiologic cause of that particular uveitic disorder associated with serous RD. Most likely, this disorder will be VKH disease, in which case high doses of systemic steroids plus another oral immunosuppressant will most likely resolve the exudative RD and causative choroidal inflammation and breakdown of retinal barrier.

References

1. Rao NA, Gupta A, Dustin L, et al. Frequency of distinguishing clinical features in Vogt-Koyanagi-Harada disease. *Ophthalmology.* 2010;117:591-599.
2. Read RW, Yu F, Accorinti M, et al. Evaluation of the effect on outcomes of the route of administration of corticosteroids in acute Vogt-Koyanagi-Harada disease. *Am J Ophthalmol.* 2006;142:119-124.
3. Paredes I, Ahmed M, Foster CS. Immunomodulatory therapy for Vogt-Koyanagi-Harada patients as first-line therapy. *Ocul Immunol Inflamm.* 2006;14:87-90.
4. Park HS, Nam KY, Kim JY. Intravitreal bevacizumab injection for persistent serous retinal detachment associated with Vogt-Koyanagi-Harada disease. *Graefes Arch Clin Exp Ophthalmol.* 2010 Aug 6. Epub ahead of print.
5. Khalifa Y, Loh AR, Acharya NR. Fluocinolone acetonide intravitreal implants in Vogt-Koyanagi-Harada disease. *Ocul Immunol Inflamm.* 2009;17:431-433.

WHAT ARE THE INDICATIONS FOR VITRECTOMY IN A PATIENT WITH UVEITIS?

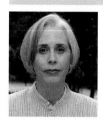

Janet L. Davis, MD

Acute inflammation in uveitis is usually efficiently controlled by high doses of topical corticosteroids in the case of anterior uveitis, or by regional or oral corticosteroids in the case of intermediate, posterior, or panuveitis. Vitrectomy in acute intraocular inflammation is probably only appropriate in selected cases of endophthalmitis or necrotizing herpetic retinitis. For uveitis persisting beyond 3 months, vitrectomy becomes a feasible tool in its management, as it may for atypical cases that fail to respond fully to corticosteroids.

Medical evidence for vitrectomy in uveitis can be categorized as clearly beneficial (A level), probably beneficial (B level), and possibly beneficial (C level); evidence for actual harm is often missing because of failure to publish. For the clinician, formal estimates of benefits translate into whether a procedure is indicated, with no or few alternatives, or elective, with clear alternatives, including other therapies or observation. In some cases, vitrectomy could be considered speculative. A compilation of published case series through 2005 reports "C" evidence levels for 44 papers including 1575 patients.[1] The studies were inconclusive because of bias in case selection, irregular follow-up, imprecise outcome measures, and lack of information on concomitant medications. No A or B level papers have been published since that time.

Vitrectomy in uveitis is indicated for the correction of posterior segment uveitic complications that otherwise meet established standards for this procedure. Common complications are epiretinal membranes with traction or recalcitrant macular edema, macular hole, retinal detachment, and nonclearing vitreous opacities. Even within this category, special circumstances of uveitis patients alter surgical planning. The need for control of inflammation pre- and postoperatively is obvious. Maculas with long-standing macular edema and poor visual prognosis may not merit either removal of epiretinal membranes or repair of macular hole. Removal of adherent membranes over cystic retina can easily lead to an intraoperative shift from peel to repair. Whereas buckling may be acceptable for many rhegmatogenous detachments in uveitis affecting the posterior segment, vitrectomy seems ideal to remove opacities and, possibly, to reduce the chance of postoperative complications, such as membrane formation. Intraoperative complications are likely increased in uveitis, including the possibility of irreparable retinal holes if instruments are passed through pars plana exudates that extend onto the retina and posterior breaks during peeling of densely adherent hyaloid and membranes from the retina, especially vessels or scars. Attention to tangential peeling rather than application of anterior-posterior forces and triamcinolone-assisted visualization of vitreous are important intraoperative maneuvers in uveitic vitrectomy. Surgery for hypotony in uveitis with ciliary body membrane stripping has been reported but is unlikely to be successful if the cause is atrophy of the ciliary processes.

The degree of vitreous opacities that warrant surgery is obviously discretionary. In general, if improvement can be anticipated with further medical treatment, the patient by definition is not adequately controlled, and surgery is not likely to accomplish the objective. On the other hand, a fully-treated, stable patient scheduled for cataract surgery who also has symptomatic vitreous opacities will not have the surgical objective of clear optical media met unless vitrectomy surgery is performed. Similarly, a post-treatment patient with nonclearing vitreous strands and debris that affect vision can be considered for therapeutic vitrectomy.

Elective indications include vitrectomy for diagnostic purposes. Both aqueous humor and vitreous can be used for polymerase chain reaction (PCR) diagnosis of infectious uveitis (eg, cytomegalovirus, herpes simplex, varicella zoster, and toxoplasmosis), especially when there is retinovascular leakage, extensive retinitis, optic nerve involvement, or immunocompromise.[2] Case series of diagnostic vitrectomies reported yields from 30% to 81.6% through 2005.[3] More recent studies have yields in the higher range. Yield is highly dependent on case selection and whether "idiopathic" is considered to be a confirmed diagnosis, but the higher-yielding series indicate that clinical judgment combined with current laboratory techniques is a viable diagnostic procedure for many cases of chorioretinitis and intraocular lymphoma. Chorioretinal biopsy is reported (and needed) in fewer cases.

The issue of elective vitrectomy as a therapeutic alternative to immunosuppressive therapy has a long history and an uncertain conclusion. It has been considered since the invention of vitrectomy, initially for pediatric uveitis during pars plana lensectomy and for endophthalmitis. The principal of vitrectomy after failure of conservative management of uveitis was formally proposed by Kaplan in 1992. There are viable scientific hypotheses that can be generated for the use of vitrectomy, including alteration of oxygen gradients by vitreous removal, increased clearance of inflammatory cells and mediators, and removal of antigens in at least some cases of occult infection. The benefits of rapid clearance should be weighed against the corollary rapid loss of therapeutic intravitreal medications, such as anti-vascular endothelial growth factor (VEGF) agents and corticosteroids.

Many of the case series of vitrectomy in uveitis propose benefits from the reduction of concomitant medical therapy or the reduction in cystoid macular edema after vitrectomy. Whereas mechanical factors of epiretinal membranes (ERM) contributing to cystoid macular edema (CME) seem highly favorable for surgical management, the benefits of removal of the cortical hyaloid because it may be trapping noxious stimuli next to the retina, or removal of the internal limiting membrane to deturgesce the Müeller cells is theoretical. Only one randomized, controlled clinical trial in patients has been attempted, which was underpowered and did not reach statistical significance.[4] Sixteen patients (20 eyes) were recruited who had active uveitis despite treatment with corticosteroids and were randomized to receive either pars plana vitrectomy or initial treatment with methotrexate. Of the 9 patients (11 eyes) randomized to pars plana vitrectomy, 8 had been removed from systemic therapy by the end of follow-up. Further study is warranted.

Clinicians who wish to use vitrectomy as the primary treatment for uveitis should follow outcomes that do not rely on simple clearing of the media and are relevant to the control of uveitis. Examples are resolution of angiographically determined retinovascular leakage in the macula and to the equator and optical coherence tomography measurements of macular thickening. Possible complications of accelerated cataract formation or worsened anterior segment inflammation should be considered, as well as the availability of a wider range of immunosuppressive medications with good safety margins. Achieving clarity of the ocular media is not equivalent to controlling uveitis. Undoubtedly, in some patients, it is the antigenic load in the vitreous or some other peculiarity of it, such as prolonged retention and preservation of lymphocytes, that perpetuates uveitis, and vitrectomy would be truly therapeutic. It has been assumed that this is the case for intermediate uveitis, but pars planitis may not be the optimal disease for vitrectomy because retinovascular leakage is so prominent. Series in Fuchs' uveitis are promising.[1] Fuchs' is now known to be a chronic viral infection, and there may be viral antigen retention in the vitreous. Vitrectomy in juvenile uveitis also appears unusually promising. This may relate to the density of vitreous in youth with even greater retention of inflammatory cells and cytokines. A case series of vitrectomy in juvenile uveitis reported improvement in the clinically relevant parameter of reduction in relapses in uveitis after vitrectomy.[5]

Summary

Vitrectomy is inevitable in some patients with uveitis who develop vitreoretinal complications. It can be used to provide ample material for diagnostic studies. As a therapy, it is promising, but ideal candidates for treatment have not been identified, and a multicenter, randomized, controlled clinical trial is likely necessary to answer the question of whether vitrectomy can serve as a primary therapy rather than as an adjunct for the management of uveitis.

References

1. Becker M, Davis J. Vitrectomy in the treatment of uveitis [Perspective]. *Am J Ophthalmol.* 2005;140:1096-1105.
2. Harper TW, Miller D, Schiffman JC, Davis JL. Polymerase chain reaction analysis of aqueous and vitreous specimens in the diagnosis of posterior segment infectious uveitis. *Am J Ophthalmol.* 2009;147:140-147.
3. Davis JL, Miller DM, Ruiz P. Diagnostic testing of vitrectomy specimens. *Am J Ophthalmol.* 2005;140:822-829.
4. Quinones K, Choi JY, Yilmaz T, Kafkala, C, Letko E, Foster CS. Pars plana vitrectomy versus immunomodulatory therapy for intermediate uveitis: a prospective, randomized pilot study. *Ocul Immunol Inflamm.* 2010;18:411-417.
5. Trittibach P, Koerner F, Sarra GM, Garweg JG. Vitrectomy for juvenile uveitis: prognostic factors for the long-term functional outcome. *Eye (London).* 2006;20:184-190.

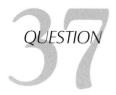

QUESTION

HOW DO YOU TREAT UVEITIS-ASSOCIATED MACULAR EDEMA?

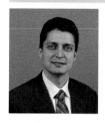

David M. Hinkle, MD

Macular edema is a leading cause of vision loss in patients with uveitis.[1] Prevention is the best form of treatment, hence the need for aggressive anti-inflammatory therapy before this potentially blinding complication develops. Gaining control of inflammation is paramount to successful therapy for uveitic macular edema. Smoking cessation is critical to the successful management of all patients with uveitis, particularly those with intermediate uveitis and macular edema.[2]

Early recognition is equally important. I use fluorescein angiography (FA) and optical coherence tomography (OCT) as complementary diagnostic tools. Some eyes have clear-cut macular leakage on the FA with minimal changes on fundus examination or OCT. In all other eyes, OCT is my preferred means of monitoring the response to treatment. The OCT pattern of macular edema may be cystoid, diffuse, or with neuroepithelial detachment. There may be poor correlation between visual acuity and retinal thickness, particularly in the first weeks following intervention.

Assuming one has eliminated active inflammation, a stepladder approach is typically employed with topical nonsteroidal anti-inflammatory agents as my first choice. Oral nonsteroidal therapy is beneficial in refractory cases provided there is no history of peptic ulcer disease. I ask patients to notify me if they develop dyspepsia and I discuss the risks of hypertension and renal damage. Either their primary care physician or I monitor blood pressure and renal function every 6 months. Acetazolamide 500 mg or less, given once daily, is beneficial in about 50% of cases.[3] If there is no response within 3 months, this should be discontinued given the potential for adverse events including dysguesia, paresthesias, electrolyte abnormalities, nephrolithiasis, and, rarely, aplastic anemia. Monthly intramuscular somatostatin injections have been successful in reports by a number of investigators.[4]

Periocular or intravitreal depot triamcinolone injection is frequently effective provided the benefit outweighs the potential risks of cataract formation or ocular hypertension for an individual patient. Periocular triamcinolone injection is my initial treatment in patients with active inflammation. The posterior sub-Tenon (Nozik technique) and inferior orbital approach are effective and carry similar risks with the exceptions that the Nozik technique carries greater risk of ptosis, whereas the inferior orbital approach carries greater risk of orbital fat prolapse. Intravitreal bevacizumab can be effective in most patients and appears to carry lower risks of cataract and glaucoma than intraocular corticosteroids.[5]

Vitrectomy with induction of posterior vitreous detachment and removal of epiretinal membrane when present is successful in one-third of refractory cases.[6] Poor prognostic factors for surgery include epiretinal membrane thickness greater than 12 µm, poor visual acuity, longer duration prior to surgery and diffuse macular edema. Long-acting intraocular steroid delivery devices can be successful when other treatment modalities have failed. Macular focal/grid photocoagulation is not effective for macular edema associated with uveitis, but peripheral retinal laser photocoagulation or cryoablation is effective in some patients with intermediate uveitis.

References

1. Rothova A, Suttorp-van Schulten MS, Frits Treffers W, Kijlstra A. Causes and frequency of blindness in patients with intraocular inflammatory disease. *Br J Ophthalmol*. 1996;80:332-336.
2. Lin P, Loh AR, Margolis TP, Acharya NR. Cigarette smoking as a risk factor for uveitis. *Ophthalmology*. 2010;117:585-590.
3. Schilling H, Heiligenhaus A, Laube T, Bornfeld N, Jurklies B. Long-term effect of acetazolamide treatment of patients with uveitic chronic cystoid macular edema is limited by persisting inflammation. *Retina*. 2005;25: 182-188.
4. Missotten T, van Laar JA, van der Loos TL, et al. Octreotide long-acting repeatable for the treatment of chronic macular edema in uveitis. *Am J Ophthalmol*. 2007;144:838-843.
5. Cordero Coma M, Sobrin L, Onal S, Christen W, Foster CS. Intravitreal bevacizumab for treatment of uveitic macular edema. *Ophthalmology*. 2007;114:1574-1579.
6. Tranos P, Scott R, Zambarakji H, Ayliffe W, Pavesio C, Charteris DG. The effect of pars plana vitrectomy on cystoid macular oedema associated with chronic uveitis: a randomised, controlled pilot study. *Br J Ophthalmol*. 2006;90:1107-1110.

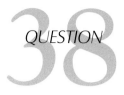

QUESTION

How Can I Differentiate Birdshot Retinochoroidopathy From the Other White Dot Syndromes?

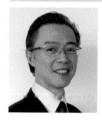

Phuc Lehoang, MD, PhD

Birdshot retinochoroidopathy (BSRC) is a rare noninfectious ocular inflammatory disease belonging to the heterogeneous group of inflammatory chorioretinopathies called white dot syndromes.

The list of diseases included in the term *white dot syndromes* (WDS) varies according to different authors. The less confusing classification is presented in the *Basic and Clinical Science Course* edited by the American Academy of Ophthalmology (Table 38-1).

Although BSRC shares some similarities with the other WDS, it represents a unique clinical entity easily identifiable based on the characteristics of its symptoms, its biomicroscopic and fundus examination, its course, and its natural history. Therefore, you need to take your time by listening to the patient's complaints and by asking the right questions. The following are some examples of questions I often ask, even before the clinical examination of the eye itself.

Questions/Answers in a Typical Case Presentation of Birdshot Retinochoroidopathy

A White 55-year-old woman with a diagnosis of uveitis comes to your clinic for blurred vision.

Q: When did you notice a visual disturbance? What kind of troubles?

143

Table 38-1

Main Inflammatory Chorioretinopathies (Previously Named White Dot Syndromes)

- Birdshot retinochoroidopathy
- Acute posterior multifocal placoid pigment epitheliopathy
- Multiple evanescent white dot syndrome
- Serpiginous choroiditis
- Multifocal choroiditis and panuveitis syndrome
- Punctate inner choroidopathy
- Subretinal fibrosis and uveitis syndrome
- Acute retinal pigment epithelitis
- Acute zonal occult outer retinopathy

A: I cannot give you an exact date of the onset but I had it for several weeks (or months), I see dark dots, specks, or spider webs moving in front of my eyes often accompanied by intermittent mobile bright lights. Those troubles are coming and going. My vision can be better when the floaters are moving out of the center of my eyes.

Interpretation: Insidious and slow progressive course, not an acute onset. The affected structures are the vitreous body with a variable degree of vitritis (floaters) and the retina (photopsia). This patient is presenting at a relatively early stage because the visual acuity seems to be only mildly affected without severe alteration of the macula or optic nerve. Chronic course with exacerbations and recurrences leads progressively to severe visual impairment. BSRC affects predominantly middle-aged patients, more frequently women than men, but can also be seen in 30- to 70-year-old patients.

Q: Which is the affected eye?
A: Both, but my left eye may be slightly worse than the right eye.

Q: Were your eyes painful and red?
A: Not at all.

Interpretation: Bilateral disease, slightly asymmetrical without acute inflammation of the anterior segment or sclera.

Q: Do you have some problems driving at night or for differentiating the colors?
A: Yes, I cannot see well when it is dark, and I am dazzled by the glare of the headlights. I mix up the colors of my clothes.

Interpretation: Nyctalopia, photophobia, color vision alteration with involvement of the retina and/or to some degree of the optic nerve.

Because the signs are bilateral, they are unlikely related to a vitreous traction with a mild intravitreal hemorrhage. Nyctalopia and color vision alteration are rarely observed during the early stages of intermediate uveitis (eg, pars planitis) but can be responsible for floaters.

At this stage, before any physical examination of the eyes, the following diagnoses encompassed by the term *white dot syndromes* are also unlikely (although the criteria are sometimes overlapping and therefore cannot be discriminating in all the cases):

- Acute posterior multifocal placoid pigment epitheliopathy (APMPPE)—Younger patient (age 20 to 50), no gender predominance, viral prodrome, frequent scotomas, no nyctalopia, no color vision disturbances.

- Multiple evanescent white dot syndrome (MEWDS)—Young female patient (age 10 to 47), acute onset, unilateral symptoms, viral prodrome in 50% of the cases, decreased visual acuity at onset, scotomas, photopsia but no nyctalopia, no color vision disturbances.

- Serpiginous choroiditis (SC)—Young and middle-aged patients (age 20 to 60); no gender predominance; bilateral but highly asymmetrical; patients present with unilateral rapidly progressive visual loss with scotomas, rare photopsia, and no nyctalopia or color vision disturbances.

- Multifocal choroiditis and panuveitis syndrome (MCP)—Younger myopic female patients (age 9 to 69), highly asymmetrical, floaters but no nyctalopia, no color vision disturbances, frequent choroidal neovascularization.

- Punctate inner choroidopathy (PIC)—Young White myopic females (age 18 to 40), asymmetric visual acuity loss with metamorphopsias, photopsias, paracentral scotomas, no vitritis, frequent choroidal neovascularization.

- Subretinal fibrosis and uveitis syndrome (SFU)—Young female patient (age 14 to 34), moderate vitritis.

- Acute retinal pigment epithelitis (ARPE)—Acute onset, mostly unilateral (75%), no vitritis, young patient (age 14 to 40), no gender predominance, no vitritis.

- Acute zonal occult outer retinopathy (AZOOR)—Young female patient (mean age 36), multiple scotomas with photopsias.

The slit-lamp and fundus examinations will provide important clues for the final diagnosis of BSRC:

- White and painless eyes.

- Minimal (fine dusty keratic precipitates) or no anterior segment inflammation. Irido-capsular synechiae are NEVER observed.

- Vitritis of variable intensity; no snow balls, no snow banking differentiating BSRC from pars planitis.

- Narrowing of the retinal arterioles.

- Distinctive, discrete, deep cream-colored or depigmented elongated oval spots scattered throughout the postequatorial fundus along the large choroidal vessels, radiating from the optic disc, more often seen in the inferior nasal area of the fundus (Figure 38-1). They measure one-quarter to three-quarters of the optic disc diameter.

It may be difficult to see those spots with a no-contact slit-lamp lens. In order to optimize the visualization of these spots, you should then try (1) to examine the fundus with a green light using a red-free filter, (2) to use a conventional indirect ophthalmoscope giving an overall view of the fundus and a better visualization of the deeper layers, (3) to take fundus red-free wide angle photographs combining the advantages of the

Figure 38-1. Color fundus photograph: elongated cream-colored spots radiating from the optic disc, following the large choroidal vessels, mostly located in the inferior nasal area.

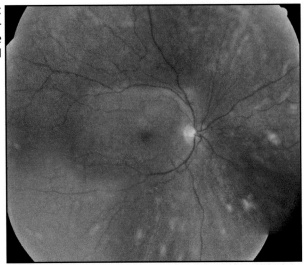

Figure 38-2. Red-free fundus picture with very few creamy spots, epiretinal membrane, and petaloid appearance of the optic disc due to birdshot spots adjacent to the papilla.

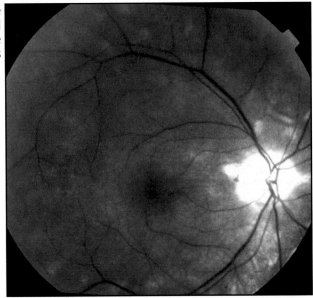

2 previous techniques. Once I have suspected a case of BSRC, I perform ancillary exams to strengthen my diagnosis and evaluate the activity of the disease and its consequences.

- Human leukocyte antigen (HLA) typing showing the presence of the HLA-A29 antigen in 90% to 100% of the cases with a relative risk above 150 is almost a diagnostic criteria, at least a strong confirmation of your hypothesis.

- Indocyanine green angiography (ICG-A): Presence of multiple hypofluorescent dots more numerous than those seen on color or red-free fundus photographs (Figures 38-2 and 38-3); they are seen at the intermediate phase of the ICG-A (between 10 and 15 minutes) and disappear during the late phase (35 to 45 minutes) in case of active choroidal granulomas.

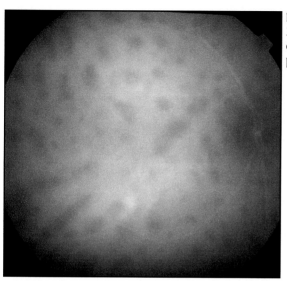

Figure 38-3. Same patient as in Figure 38-3; numerous scattered hypofluorescent dots revealed during the intermediate phase of the ICG-A.

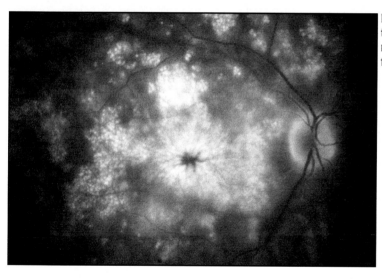

Figure 38-4. Diffuse cystoid edema of the posterior pole (late stage of the fluorescein angiogram).

- The fluorescein angiograms (FA) do not highlight the cream-colored spots but can show retinal vascular leakage, hyperfluorescence of the optic disc, and cystoid macular edema complicating a longstanding active intraocular inflammation (Figure 38-4).
- Visual field alterations can inaugurate the disease or be observed with extended follow-up along with electroretinogram abnormalities (decrease in b-wave amplitude, delay in the 30-Hz flicker implicit time) suggesting diffuse retinal dysfunction.
- Evaluation of macular changes by optical coherence tomography (OCT) examination (edema, epiretinal membrane).

Once you have performed most of these investigations and know the history of your patient, you will be able to exclude the differential diagnosis, which will have important implications in terms of management.

Other White Dot Syndromes

- APMPPE—Acute multifocal, flat gray lesions, larger than the Birdshot lesions (1 to 2 disc areas), early blockage and late staining on FA, hypofluorescent spots on ICG-A; good prognosis.

- MEWDS—Unilateral; very mild anterior uveitis and vitritis, small evanescent perifoveal white-orange dots (100 to 200 µm), granular pigment changes of macula; enlarged blind spot and scotomas; FA: early punctate hyperfluorescence with late staining; ICG-A: hypofluorescent dots more numerous than the ones seen on clinical examination or on FA. Good prognosis with spontaneous restoration of the vision within 1 to 3 months.

- SC—Geographic large, yellowish chorioretinal lesions at the posterior pole and around the optic disc with pronounced opacification at the edges of the lesions leading to chorioretinal atrophy; frequent macular choroidal neovascularization; FA: early hypofluorescence with late hyperfluorescence of the active borders; ICG-A: early hypofluorescence, late staining involving a larger area than the one seen on color pictures or on FA; guarded prognosis.

- MCP—Anterior uveitis (50%); vitritis (100%); small yellowish chorioretinal lesions evolving to punched-out scars (50 to 200 µm) often extend to the midperiphery; optic disc edema, peripapillary pigment changes; frequent macular choroidal neovascularization; guarded prognosis.

- PIC—No vitritis; frequent macular choroidal neovascularization.

- SFU—Large stellate zones of subretinal fibrosis, 50 to 500 µm yellow-white lesions; visual field, ERG, EOG profound attenuation.

- ARPE—Small hyperpigmented lesions with a yellow halo at the posterior pole, normal ERG, abnormal EOG, excellent prognosis.

- AZOOR—Large zones of outer retinal function loss with minimal funduscopic changes, subtle RPE atrophy, focal perivenous sheathing, diffuse hyperfluorescence at the late stages of the fluorescein angiogram, abnormal ERG and visual fields.

Other chorioretinopathies, although often easy to rule out, you must always keep in mind the following differential diagnosis:
Mostly noninfectious:
- Sarcoidosis
- Vogt-Koyanagi-Harada syndrome (VKH)
- Sympathetic ophthalmia
- Intraocular lymphoma, mucosal-associated lymphoid tissue
Infectious:
- Tuberculosis
- Syphilis
- Ocular histoplasmosis syndrome
- Diffuse unilateral subacute neuroretinitis (DUSN)
- Toxoplasmosis
- Pneumocystis choroidopathy

Course: You may be faced with an advanced-stage disease suffering from a progressive chronic intraocular inflammation with choroiditis, retinal vasculitis, cystoid macular edema, and optic nerve inflammation constantly leading to severe visual loss and late complications including optic and retinal atrophy with major pigment changes, atrophic scarring of the birdshot lesions, epiretinal membranes, and exceptional choroidal neovascularization.

The treatment of BSRC must be administered early in the course of the disease to prevent severe visual loss secondary to a continuous and progressive course generally marked by multiple exacerbations leading to irreversible damage of the retina and the optic nerve. Systemic corticosteroid monotherapy by itself is not sufficient to control the disease in the long term. Immunomodulatory therapy is required and is often the first line of therapy.

Summary

In most cases, in order to make the diagnosis of BSRC you only need the following:
- A simple but complete documented patient's medical history (ask the right questions).

- A careful clinical examination without forgetting the conventional indirect ophthalmoscopy.

- A confirmation by the presence of the HLA-A29 antigen.

The other ancillary tests are mandatory to manage and monitor the treatment.

Suggested Readings

American Academy of Ophthalmology, ed. *Basic and Clinical Science Course (BCSC)*. San Francisco, CA: Author; 2009-2010:183-186.

LeHoang P, Ryan SJ. Birdshot retinochoroidopathy. In: Pepose JS, Holland GN, Wilhelmus KR, eds. *Ocular Infection and Immunity*. St. Louis, MO: Mosby-Year Book Inc; 1996:570-578.

Nussenblatt RB, Whitcup SM. White-dot syndromes. In: Nussenblatt RB, Whitcup SM, eds. *Uveitis, Fundamentals and Clinical Practice*. Philadelphia, PA: Mosby-Elsevier; 2010:383-400.

Opremcak EM. Birdshot retinochoroiditis. In: Albert DM, Jakobiec FA, eds. *Principles and Practice of Ophthalmology*. Philadelphia, PA: WB Saunders; 1994:475-480.

Ryan SJ, Maumenee AE. Birdshot retinochoroidopathy. *Am J Ophthalmol*. 1980;89:31-45.

Shah KH, Levinson RD, Yu F, et al. Birdshot chorioretinopathy. *Surv Ophthalmol*. 2005;50:519-541.

Vitale AT. Birdshot retinochoroidopathy. In Foster CS, Vitale AT, eds. *Diagnosis and Treatment of Uveitis*. Philadelphia, PA: WB Saunders; 2002:731-741.

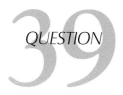

QUESTION

39

DOES B-SCAN ULTRASONOGRAPHY ASSIST IN EVALUATING A PATIENT WITH UVEITIS?

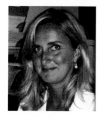

Elisabetta Miserocchi, MD

Ultrasonography (US) is a noninvasive imaging technique that can help the uveitis specialist in the differential diagnosis of various types of intraocular and periocular inflammatory diseases. Ophthalmic US employs high-frequency sound waves that provide the high resolution required for ocular diagnosis. The main advantages of this method are that it is relatively inexpensive, rapid, produces images in real time, can obtain images in different planes (changing rapidly from one plane to another one), and does not produce biologic hazards. The disadvantages are the need for direct contact with the globe or eyelid (that make examination impossible in the case of acute pain) and the dependence on operator skills.

In the diagnosis of posterior scleritis, US is the most helpful ancillary test in detecting posterior inflammation of the sclera. The hallmark features of posterior scleritis seen with B-mode US are helpful in differentiating posterior scleritis from other conditions. Fluid can accumulate in the posterior episcleral space and extend around the optic nerve, forming the characteristic "T-sign" on B-scan (Figure 39-1). B-scan US may reveal the characteristic flattening of the posterior aspect of the globe due to retrobulbar edema. Abnormally increased thickening of the posterior ocular surface of the globe more than 2 mm, optic disc swelling, distension of the optic nerve sheath, retinal detachments, and choroidal detachments can be detected.[1]

US may help in visualization of the posterior segment in patients with diffuse posterior synechia. This is particularly true for children with juvenile idiopathic arthritis-associated uveitis. Fundus examination in those young patients is already very difficult in the setting of an outpatient clinic, in particular when there are strong synechia between the iris and the lens that hamper an appropriate visualization of the

Figure 39-1. Characteristic T-sign on B-scan US in case of posterior scleritis.

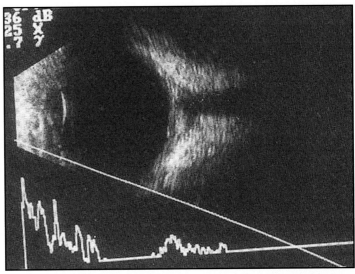

Figure 39-2. Typical mushroom shape in choroidal melanoma.

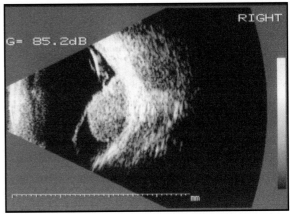

posterior pole. Echography can be a quick and noninvasive tool to detect signs of posterior pole involvement (vitritis, retinal detachment, optic disc edema, presence of snow bank suggestive of pars planitis).

Echography may be of interest in the work-up of Vogt-Koyanagi-Harada when the media are opacified or pupillary dilatation is difficult. It can show thickening of the posterior choroid and serous retinal detachments. Echography is, however, not sufficient to detect subtle intrachoroidal inflammatory lesions.[2]

US may help in the differential diagnosis of masquerade syndromes. Choroidal melanoma (choroidal and ciliary body melanomas) may present with significant posterior uveitis. These cases may be very similar to the presentation of sarcoid, tuberculous uveitis, or posterior scleritis, and the choroidal mass may be misdiagnosed as a granuloma. B-scan US combined with A-scan has a more than 95% accuracy in the diagnosis of choroidal melanoma more than 3 mm thick. The characteristic features on B-scan are an acoustically silent zone within the melanoma, choroidal excavation, and the typical mushroom shape with low-medium internal reflectivity and lack of halo (Figure 39-2).[3]

Patients with retinal vasculitis may require US for diagnosis and follow-up of vitreous hemorrhages. The most common inflammatory retinal disease that complicates vitreous hemorrhages and secondary tractional retinal detachment is Eale disease. Eale disease is an idiopathic, usually peripheral, bilateral retinal vasculitis resulting in peripheral non-perfusion and neovascularization in young otherwise healthy males.[4]

Systemic autoimmune diseases, such as Wegener's granulomatosis, can manifest with myositis. In myositis, there is usually a diffuse thickening of the involved muscle, including the inserting tendon to the globe with echolucency on B-scan and low reflectivity on A-scan. Comparative assessment with other muscles, especially the counterpart of the other orbit, is quite revealing for the condition.

B-scan US can help in the differential diagnosis of inflammatory optic disc edema, papillitis, or optic disc drusen.[5]

Retained intraocular foreign body can cause various degrees of inflammation leading to persistent anterior or posterior uveitis. The inflammatory feature secondary to an intraocular foreign body may masquerade as uveitis. B-scan US can give a general idea of the presence and relative position of an intraocular foreign body and will be especially useful in eyes with small particles, opaque media, poor patient cooperation, or hidden location.[6]

References

1. Foster CS, Sainz de la Maza M. *The Sclera*. New York, NY: Springer-Verlag; 1994.
2. Forster DJ, Cano MR, Green RL, Rao NA. Echographic features of the Vogt Koyanagi-Harada syndrome. *Arch Ophthalmol*. 1990;108:1421-1426.
3. Read RW, Zamir E, Rao NA. Neoplastic masquerade syndromes. *Surv Ophthalmol*. 2002;47:81-124.
4. Biswas J, Sharma T, Gopal L, et al. Eales' disease—an update. *Surv Ophthalmol*. 2002;47:197-214.
5. Kurz-Levin MM, Landau K. A comparison of imaging techniques for diagnosing drusen of the optic nerve head. *Arch Ophthalmol*. 1999;117:1045-1049.
6. Waheed NK, Young LH. Intraocular foreign body related endophthalmitis. *Int Ophthalmol Clin*. 2007;47:165-171.

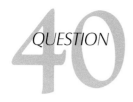

WHEN SHOULD I ORDER FLUORESCEIN ANGIOGRAPHY OR OCULAR COHERENCE TOMOGRAPHY IN A PATIENT WITH UVEITIS?

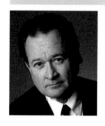

E. Mitchel Opremcak, MD

Fluorescein angiography (FA) and ocular coherence tomography (OCT) can be very useful tests in the evaluation and treatment of patients with uveitis. Both FA and OCT require a degree of media clarity and are unable to be used in patients with dense cataract or significant vitreous opacification, which is often the case in patients with uveitis.

Fluorescein angiography provides photographic imaging of the retinal and choroidal circulations and the status of the retinal blood-eye-barriers (BEBs). The fluorescein molecule is normally confined to within the retinal vessels via tight junctions between the vascular endothelial cells and to the choroid via tight junctions between healthy and intact retinal pigment epithelial cells (RPE). Inflammation often results in a breakdown of these tight junctions and results in fluorescein extravasation. OCT provides a sagittal image of the macular architecture from the retinal surface to the choroid.[1] OCT is quickly performed and is noninvasive. FA and OCT complement each other, and I use them in my uveitis patients to help in 1) establishing a diagnosis, 2) assessing sequelae of uveitis, 3) determining response to therapy, and 4) in patients with unexplained vision loss.

Fluorescein Angiography

FA is often used to help diagnose many of the "white dot syndromes" of the retina. Active lesions in acute posterior multifocal placoid pigment epitheliopathy (APMPPE) and punctate inner choroiditis (PIC) will have a "block early and stain late" pattern.[2] Multiple

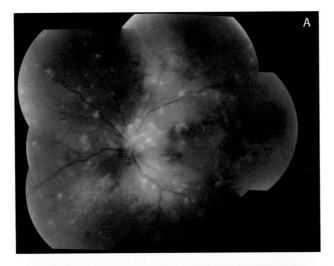

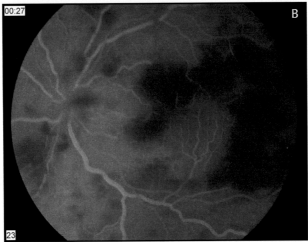

Figure 40-1. (A) Fundus photograph of a patient with retinal vasculitis. (B) The fluorescein angiogram demonstrating inflammation of the venules.

evanescent white dot syndrome (MEWDS) will have a characteristic "wreath sign," and birdshot retinochoroidopathy (BRC) lesions are often unimpressive on FA. I will also use FA in determining whether a retinal vasculitis primarily involves the arterioles or venules (Figure 40-1). Inflamed retinal arterioles or venules will demonstrate fluorescein dye staining, indicating a breakdown of the BEB. Arterioles are primarily affected in certain disorders, such as acute retinal necrosis syndrome (ARN), while venules are involved in BRC and Behçet's disease.

The sequelae of severe intraocular inflammation include retinal edema, capillary nonperfusion, neovascularization, and breakdown of the BEB and can all be documented with FA. Choroidal nonperfusion can be seen in systemic lupus erythematosus (SLE) and giant cell arteritis and may be a component of the hypofluorescence seen in APMPPE. Choroidal neovascularization (CNV) can be found in virtually any posterior uveitis syndrome. CNV is very common in ocular histoplasmosis syndrome,

PIC, and even in serpiginous choroiditis.[3] Treatment with newer anti-vascular endothelial growth factor agents can be considered and has been met with much success. Breakdown of the BEB at the level of the RPE can be found in Vogt-Koyanagi-Harada syndrome, posterior scleritis, and syphilis. The characteristic multifocal, punctate, hyperfluorescent lesions and secondary pooling of the fluorescein dye in these angiograms help me with my differential diagnosis. Cystoid macular edema (CME) can be found in all forms of uveitis. FA will demonstrate the classic petaloid appearance within the sensory retina. Retinal vasculitis, capillary nonperfusion, and retinal neovascularization are commonly seen in patients with SLE and Behçet's disease. I use the angiogram to determine the extent of capillary nonperfusion, which then guides any necessary laser photoablation.

FA can be used to follow response to therapy. As an example, patients with BRC will often present with severe CME and retinal vasculitis. These patients will often respond to initial corticosteroid therapies and subsequent, maintenance-immunomodulatory therapy. FA will demonstrate any resolution of the CME and vasculitis and any remaining edema requiring additional treatment.

In my uveitis patients with unexplained loss of visual acuity, FA can be very helpful in determining the cause. FA may find occult CNV, subtle CME, or mild capillary nonperfusion that was unrecognized on biomicroscopy.

Ocular Coherence Tomography

While OCT is rarely diagnostic for any specific uveitis syndrome, I find that I am using OCT more often than FA in my uveitis patients. OCT is rapid, noninvasive, and can provide near histological information at micron resolution in the posterior pole and macula. As a result, if I am looking for certain sequelae such as CME, macular hole, fixed macular cysts, vitreomacular traction (VMT), or an epiretinal membrane (ERM), the OCT will quickly provide this information. In many cases, the OCT is superior to FA in demonstrating CME, ERM, and VMT. OCT can also demonstrate subretinal fluid (SRF) from an exudative retinal detachment (Vogt-Koyanagi-Harada syndrome; VKH) or CNV (presumed ocular histoplasmosis syndrome; POHS). The OCT is more sensitive than FA in demonstrating very subtle amounts of SRF in these cases.

While FA can be used to follow treatment response, the convenience of the OCT makes it the study of choice when following resolution of CME or treatment responses for a CNV. The OCT can be performed at 4- to 6-week intervals following periocular, intraocular, or systemic therapies to determine the need for additional or more aggressive treatments.

I will often start with an OCT in my patients with unexplained visual loss. When biomicroscopy fails to show a reason for vision loss, the OCT can show even subtle amounts of SRF, CME, ERM, or VMT (Figure 40-2). Significant thinning and atrophy of the macula may also result in loss of vision in patients with end-stage BRC and in Behçet's disease. OCT can demonstrate this sensory retinal atrophy and help explain the loss of vision.

Figure 40-2. OCT showing vitreomacular traction.

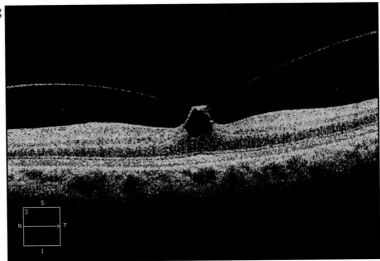

References

1. Mirza, RG, Johnson MW, Jampol LM. Optical coherence tomography use in evaluation of the vitreoretinal interface: a review. *Surv Ophthalmol*. 2007;52:397.
2. Gass JD. Acute posterior multifocal placoid pigment epitheliopathy. *Arch Ophthalmol*. 1968;80:177.
3. Jampol LM, Orth D, Daily MJ, Raab MF. Subretinal neovascularization with geographic (serpiginous) choroiditis. *Am J Ophthalmol*. 1979;88:683.

WHAT IS THE RISK OF STERILITY IN PATIENTS WITH UVEITIS WHO REQUIRE IMMUNOMODULATORY THERAPY?

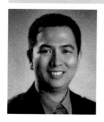

Manolette R. Roque, MD, MBA

Steroid-sparing immunomodulatory therapy, which includes antimetabolites (eg, aza-thioprine or methotrexate), alkylating agents (eg, cyclophosphamide or chlorambucil), calcineurin inhibitors (eg, cyclosporine), and biologic response modifiers (eg, infliximab, daclizumab, rituximab, adalimumab or intravenous immunoglobulin [IVIG]), is used in the treatment of patients with uveitis. The solid evidence of the success of immunomodu-latory therapy in managing uveitis is often overshadowed by the inappropriate fear of both physicians and patients regarding its associated complications. Immunomodulatory therapy has always had a bad reputation when it comes to its double-edged manner of providing a cure to cancer. As is true in daily life, first impressions do appear to last for-ever. In this regard, immunomodulatory therapy takes no exception to this generalization and falls victim to its ill repute even when used for treatment of patients with uveitis. With its use in uveitis at a fraction of the doses required for cancer treatment notwithstanding, the perception remains as notorious and unforgiving. We, therefore, have additional chal-lenges in convincing others about the rationale for its use. One of the foremost concerns raised by my colleagues and patients would be the risk of sterility attendant to the use of immunomodulatory therapy. Is the risk real? If so, is it significant? In order to justify my response, I have searched the literature for reports on the risk of sterility in patients who require immunomodulatory therapy. The following is what is reported in the literature.

Antimetabolites

In a case series of 160 patients on methotrexate for chronic noninfectious uveitis, there was no report of sterility as a side effect or adverse reaction.[1]

Eighty-four consecutive patients with inflammatory eye disease treated with mycophenolate mofetil at an academic referral center revealed gastrointestinal upset, elevated liver enzyme levels, and cytopenias but no sterility.[2]

T-Cell Inhibitor

A nonrandomized retrospective case-series study analyzing cyclosporine in the treatment of 28 eyes with Behçet's from a single uveitis center revealed mild morbidity but no gonadal dysfunction.[3]

A retrospective clinical case series of 118 eyes using oral low-dose cyclosporine for the management of sight-threatening uveitis at an academic referral center revealed a manageable toxicity profile without gonadal dysfunction.[4]

Alkylating Agents

Sterility is a major concern related to chlorambucil and to cyclophosphamide therapy.

In a noncomparative interventional case series of 56 eyes, men are seemingly more susceptible to sterility than women. A relationship has been described between cumulative dose of therapy and gonadal effect of chlorambucil. It has been shown that cumulative doses less than 8.2 mg/kg in children and 6.1 mg/kg in adults do not affect fertility.[5]

A nonrandomized retrospective case-series study analyzing chlorambucil in the treatment of 26 patients with Behçet's from a single uveitis center showed a staggering 35.7% with gonadal dysfunction.[6]

Cyclophosphamide is a known teratogen and causes sterility in both men and women beyond certain cumulative doses. Fairley and associates observed gonadal dysfunction in 60% of patients after 6 months of treatment with cyclophosphamide. They reported that Cytoxan in daily doses of 50 to 100 mg had produced low sperm counts and azoospermia in 31 men. Cytoxan therapy before puberty has been found to induce permanent sterility in males but not in females. However, in controlled studies, Cytoxan (75 mg per square meter) does not cause sterility if given only for 8 weeks. Preliminary observations indicate that a second or third course of Cytoxan therapy for 8 weeks appears to be safe.[7]

More recently, Martin et al reported premature menopause to occur in 0% to 20% of patients on IV cyclophosphamide therapy.[7] This number is substantially decreased with the concomitant administration of gonadotropin-releasing hormone therapy. As an additional precautionary measure, all males of reproductive age should be advised to bank their sperm before initiating cyclophosphamide therapy.

Tumor Necrosis Factor Inhibitor

Studies evaluating chemotherapy for ocular inflammatory disease showed an increased risk for cancer but not sterility found in infliximab.

Summary

These are a few of the numerous reports on the side effects, sterility in particular, of immunomodulatory therapy. Even though the use of immunomodulatory therapy is associated with potential side effects, most immunomodulatory therapy does not induce sterility. The risk of sterility in patients with uveitis who require immunomodulatory therapy is low to absent unless alkylating agents are used. The evidence suggests that the use of alkylating agents is the only immunomodulatory therapy that can cause gonadal dysfunction.

Today, it is possible to safely bank sperm or eggs or induce menopause before initiation of alkylating agents. With the option of sperm cryopreservation now readily available, I believe that sterility is a risk worth taking in the quest to prevent blindness in patients with uveitis, in the event that alkylating therapy is the only treatment option available for saving sight.

References

1. Samson CM, Waheed N, Baltatzis S, Foster CS. Methotrexate therapy for chronic noninfectious uveitis. Analysis of a case series of 160 patients. *Ophthalmology.* 2001;108:1134-1139.
2. Thorne JE, Jabs DA, Qazi FA, Nguyen QD, Kempen JH, Dunn JP. Mycophenolate mofetil therapy for inflammatory eye disease. *Ophthalmology.* 2005;112:1472-1477.
3. Mathews D, Mathews J, Jones NP. Low-dose cyclosporine treatment for sight-threatening uveitis: efficacy, toxicity, and tolerance. *Indian J Ophthalmol.* 2010;58:55-58.
4. Zaghetto JM, Yamamoto MM, Souza MB, et al. Chlorambucil and cyclosporine A in Brazilian patients with Behçet's disease uveitis—a retrospective study. *Arq Bras Oftalmol.* 2010;73:40-46.
5. Miserocchi E, Baltatzis S, Ekong A, Roque M, Foster CS. Efficacy and safety of chlorambucil in intractable noninfectious uveitis: the Massachusetts Eye and Ear Infirmary experience. *Ophthalmology.* 2002;109:137-142.
6. Fairley KF, Barrie JU, Johnson W. Sterility and testicular atrophy related to cyclophosphamide therapy. *Lancet.* 1972;1:568-569.
7. Martin F, Lauwerys B, Lefebvre C, et al. Side effects of intravenous cyclophosphamide pulse therapy. *Lupus.* 1997;6:254-257.

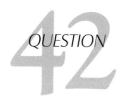

QUESTION

42

How Do the Results of the Systemic Immunosuppressive Therapy for Eye Diseases Cohort Study Apply to the Care of My Patients With Uveitis?

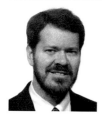

John H. Kempen, MD, PhD

Consider a patient with severe, chronic, noninfectious uveitis or scleritis whose vision is threatened when the disease is active, but who suffers a reactivation each time prednisone is tapered below 20 mg/day. Such a patient is in a bind between ocular damage and visual loss, and the certainty of severe systemic complications if corticosteroids are not tapered further. While progress is being made in developing local drug delivery alternatives to the chronic corticosteroid therapy, the best-attested approach to such a case is to apply the lessons learned decades ago in rheumatology: make use of corticosteroid-sparing drugs to solve the patient's problem. Guidelines for the use of these drugs in the setting of ophthalmology are available,[1] uveitis specialists are increasingly available to help implement the treatment, and in places where uveitis specialists are not yet available, rheumatologists can help apply the treatment. Nevertheless, recent data suggest these approaches are not being widely used,[2] which likely has severe consequences for patients overtreated with systemic corticosteroids. Perhaps clinicians and patients behave this way because of fears that immunosuppressive drugs will cause long-term side effects, such as cancer and death. To address this concern, my colleagues and I have conducted the Systemic Immunosuppressive Therapy for Eye Diseases (SITE) Cohort Study, a systematic effort to document the risks and benefits of immunosuppressive therapy for eye diseases.

First, we conducted a comprehensive evaluation of the literature as to whether the existing reports—mostly from rheumatologic, transplant, and other systemic disease cohorts—do or do not suggest that an increased risk of cancer in fact exists.[3] We found that the evidence did not support a clinically important increase in the risk of cancer with the immunosuppressive drugs most commonly used for management of eye diseases—methotrexate and mycophenolate mofetil. Reports regarding the older drug methotrexate were particularly robust. The transplant literature suggests that cancer risk in major organ transplant patients is higher with cyclosporine and possibly azathioprine than with mycophenolate mofetil; however, in the literature regarding nontransplant patients, increased risk of cancer with these agents is not particularly evident. Given the results of part 2 of the SITE Cohort Study (see below), it is likely that these drugs interact with the highly oncogenic setting of the transplant patient in a way that is mostly likely not relevant for ocular inflammation patients. In contrast, the available evidence clearly supports the oncogenicity of alkylating agents (cyclophosphamide and chlorambucil) when used in a manner that overlaps the most common approach to treating ocular inflammation.[1] The majority of the reports supported no increased risk of cancer with tumor necrosis factor (TNF)-inhibitors (eg, infliximab, adalimumab, and etanercept); although, there was one concerning exception: the extent of information in favor of no increased cancer risk with TNF-inhibitors in the rheumatoid arthritis setting is impressive.

The major limitation of this review was that most data did not derive from ocular inflammation patients, who might differ in the risk and treatment patterns. Hence, part 2 of the SITE effort was to assess the long-term risks of these agents in an ocular inflammation cohort. A large cohort of approximately 8000 patients seen between 1979 and 2005 was assembled from 5 tertiary United States ocular inflammation subspecialty centers and was followed for the occurrence of death, and death specifically due to cancer.[4] Among these patients, about 25% had taken immunosuppressive drugs. These results (Figures 42-1 and 42-2) confirmed that the most commonly used immunosuppressive drugs (the antimetabolites methotrexate, mycophenolate mofetil, and azathioprine and the T-cell inhibitor cyclosporine) were not associated with an increased risk of death, with risk ratios typically less than or equal to 1.0. The overall risk of mortality with alkylating agents was 1.17-fold higher than among patients who did not receive immunosuppressive drugs (95% confidence interval [CI]: 0.85 to 1.61), and the risk of death due to cancer was 1.74-fold higher (95% CI: 0.91 to 3.32). While neither of these results was statistically significant, the results interpreted in light of the literature review leave me with concerns that intermediate- to long-term use of alkylating agents does increase the risk of cancer to a degree that constrains their use to the most severe cases of ocular inflammation. All of these results were robust to a wide variety of sensitivity analyses, and no subset (eg, patients receiving higher doses) was observed to have higher or lower risk.

Patients who had received TNF-inhibitors were relatively few in number, and 74% of them had systemic inflammatory diseases, which may themselves predispose to cancer and early death. These patients had a marginally significant elevated increased risk of both overall (relative risk = 1.99, 95% CI: 1.00 to 3.98) and cancer mortality (relative risk = 3.83, 95% CI: 1.13 to 13.01). Given the favorable results vis-à-vis cancer with these drugs in rheumatoid arthritis patients, I think that these results may reflect the effects of the systemic diseases for which these patients were being treated, rather than treatment effects (we had insufficient observations to analyze results in patients free of systemic disease). More information about this issue is clearly needed.

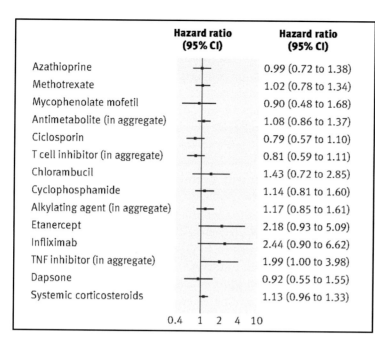

Figure 42-1. Adjusted relative hazard of all-cause mortality for each immunosuppressive agent and class of agents studied. (Reprinted with permission from Kempen JH, Daniel E, Dunn JP, et al. Overall and cancer related mortality among patients with ocular inflammation treated with immunosuppressive drugs: retrospective cohort study. *BMJ*. 2009;339:b2480.)

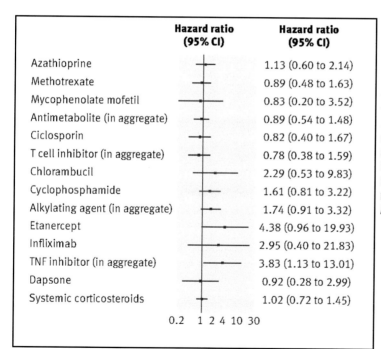

Figure 42-2. Adjusted relative hazard of mortality attributed to cancer for each immunosuppressive agent and class of agents studied. (Reprinted with permission from Kempen JH, Daniel E, Dunn JP, et al. Overall and cancer related mortality among patients with ocular inflammation treated with im-munosuppressive drugs: retrospective cohort study. *BMJ*. 2009;339:b2480.)

The third part of the study was to assess the benefits of immunosuppressive therapies for eye diseases.[5-9] These results are too complex to review in detail here, but the gist of the results was that the agents work, although not in every case, and often only after several months. Cyclophosphamide had the unique property that the majority of patients able to tolerate a full course of therapy were able to stop the drug because of disease remission, which was infrequently seen with the other agents. The ability to cause remission likely applies to chlorambucil as well. In general, most patients were able to tolerate the drugs, but 10% to 17.5% of patients taking methotrexate, mycophenolate mofetil, or cyclosporine stopped treatment within 1 year because of reversible short-term toxicities; cessation due to short-term toxicity was higher with azathioprine (23%) and cyclophosphamide (33.5%).

These results provide a great degree of reassurance that use of methotrexate, mycophenolate mofetil, azathioprine, and cyclosporine is generally safe in patients with ocular inflammation, certainly safer than long-term use of high-dose prednisone. Alkylating agents seem to have a clinically important risk of inducing cancer, but I believe they have a role in the tertiary management of highly blinding eye diseases, especially considering their potentially curative properties. In training, many ophthalmologists seem to think the classic "step ladder" approach to management of ocular inflammation means that immunosuppressive drugs are more dangerous and more effective than systemic corticosteroids. This is the wrong message: we use immunosuppressive drugs typically because they are safer, not because they are more effective than high-dose corticosteroids (hence the "corticosteroid-sparing" concept). I hope that these strong results supporting the safety and effectiveness of these agents will overcome hesitation among my colleagues and their patients in using them when they are indicated.

References

1. Jabs DA, Rosenbaum JT, Foster CS, et al. Guidelines for the use of immunosuppressive drugs in patients with ocular inflammatory disorders: recommendations of an expert panel. *Am J Ophthalmol.* 2000;130:492-513.
2. Nguyen QD, Hatef E, Kayen B, et al. A cross-sectional study of the current treatment patterns in noninfectious uveitis among specialists in the United States. *Ophthalmology.* 2011;118:184-190. Epub 2010 Aug 3.
3. Kempen JH, Gangaputra S, Daniel E, et al. Long-term risk of malignancy among patients treated with immunosuppressive agents for ocular inflammation: a critical assessment of the evidence. *Am J Ophthalmol.* 2008;146:802-812.
4. Kempen JH, Daniel E, Dunn JP, et al. Overall and cancer related mortality among patients with ocular inflammation treated with immunosuppressive drugs: retrospective cohort study. *BMJ.* 2009;339:b2480.
5. Pujari SS, Kempen JH, Newcomb CW, et al. Cyclophosphamide for ocular inflammatory diseases. *Ophthalmology.* 2010;117:356-365.
6. Kacmaz RO, Kempen JH, Newcomb C, et al. Cyclosporine for ocular inflammatory diseases. *Ophthalmology.* 2009;117:576-584.
7. Daniel E, Thorne JE, Newcomb CW, et al. Mycophenolate mofetil for ocular inflammation. *Am J Ophthalmol.* 2010;149:423-432.
8. Gangaputra S, Newcomb CW, Liesegang TL, et al. Methotrexate for ocular inflammatory diseases. *Ophthalmology.* 2009;116:2188-2198.
9. Pasadhika S, Kempen JH, Newcomb CW, et al. Azathioprine for ocular inflammatory diseases. *Am J Ophthalmol.* 2009;148:500-509.

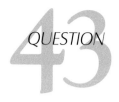
HOW LONG SHOULD I WAIT TO PERFORM CATARACT SURGERY ONCE AN EYE WITH UVEITIS IS INFLAMMATION FREE?

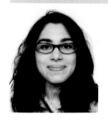

Sarah Syeda, BSc(MedSci)
(co-authored with Ellen N. Yu, MD)

Cataracts develop in the uveitic eye secondary to chronic inflammation or as a consequence of long-term treatment with corticosteroids or cholinergic antiglaucoma medications. The incidence in many forms of uveitis approaches 50%, while it is more frequent in Fuchs' heterochromic iridocyclitis and juvenile idiopathic arthritis (JIA).

Cataract extraction in uveitic eyes is not as straightforward as in nonuveitic eyes and may be associated with blinding complications if meticulous control of inflammation is not obtained prior to performing surgery and in the postoperative period. Loss of vision has been reported to occur postoperatively in about 10% of uveitic patients after cataract surgery,[1] which emphasizes the greater potential for complications in these eyes.

The 4 main indications for cataract surgery in patients with uveitis are 1) phacogenic uveitis, 2) visual impairment secondary to cataract with preoperative control of inflammation and expected good visual prognosis, 3) cataract that impairs fundus assessment and treatment in suspected fundus pathology, and 4) cataract that obstructs visualization of the posterior segment in a patient requiring posterior segment surgery.[2]

Except for phacogenic uveitis, which requires urgent surgical intervention to remove the leaking lens protein that causes intraocular inflammation, there should be an inflammation-free period of at least 3 months prior to cataract surgery for all other causes of uveitis. This may occur spontaneously for relapsing and remittent uveitis in remission or may require the use of immunomodulatory therapy or short-term corticosteroids in chronic cases. The aim is to keep the eyes inflammation free before, during, and after cataract extraction to avoid complications and ensure best visual outcome.

Preoperative Control of Inflammation

Regular preoperative examination should be performed to ensure a quiet eye for at least 3 months prior to surgery, especially those with aggressive disease such as JIA-associated uveitis and Behçet's disease. In Behçet's disease, it has even been recommended that surgery be postponed until at least 6 months of quiescence to reduce the chance of postoperative inflammation.[3]

Accurate diagnosis of uveitis is essential for management and prognostication. Some forms of infectious uveitis, such as recurrent herpetic uveitis and ocular toxoplasmosis (particularly those with lesions in the macular area or the optic nerve), warrant prophylactic antibiotic use due to a tendency for recurrence after cataract surgery.

For autoimmune uveitis, prophylactic use of anti-inflammatory agents 3 to 7 days preoperatively may be considered with topical prednisone acetate 1% 6 times a day, oral prednisone at 1 mg/kg/day, or local injections.

A careful posterior segment examination is necessary for patient selection to rule out pathologies that would hinder improvement of visual acuity after surgery. Pre-existing cystoid macular edema (CME), choroiditis, optic neuropathy, and retinal/choroidal neovascularization or detachment affects the visual outcome, and the patient should be informed beforehand. Ocular ultrasound must be performed if there is no view of the posterior pole.

Intraoperative Techniques

Surgical planning is important in the surgery of the uveitic cataract. Additional surgical steps, such as synechiolysis, insertion of iris hooks or dilator, the use of tryphan blue for capsular staining, aspiration of bleeding iris or angle vessels, and intravitreal injection of medications may be necessary. Phacoemulsification is preferred over extracapsular cataract extraction as it decreases the incidence of postoperative inflammation. Acrylic lenses provide the lowest levels of early inflammation with a reduced incidence of posterior capsular opacification (PCO) and CME. Some authors do not recommend the use of hydrophilic lenses due to accelerated PCO formation. At major risk for intraocular lens (IOL) intolerance are intermediate uveitis, panuveitis, JIA, and resistant chronic uveitis such as sarcoidosis.[4]

Other intraoperative measures include intravitreal triamcinolone acetate to reduce postoperative inflammation and CME, but these carry the risk of increased intraocular pressure (IOP) and PCO and should not be used in eyes with a history of glaucoma or steroid-responsive ocular hypertension.

Postoperative Management

The mainstay of postoperative management includes topical corticosteroids and antibiotics as well as continuation of immunomodulatory therapy. Common postoperative complications include PCO, CME, postoperative inflammation, and posterior synechiae

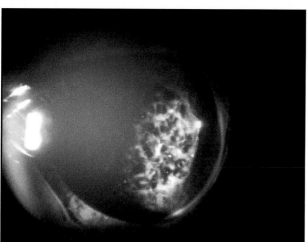

Figure 43-1. Inflammatory membrane behind the intraocular lens in a post-capsulotomy eye with poorly controlled uveitis

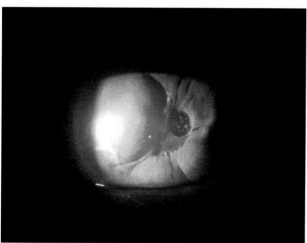

Figure 43-2. Pupillary membrane, posterior synechiae, pigment and inflammatory cell deposition on the lens surface, iris bombe, and elevation of intraocular pressure in a uveitic eye with intraocular lens intolerance.

(Figures 43-1 and 43-2), and may be prevented with aggressive perioperative control of inflammation. The incidence of CME is significantly reduced in patients who have been ocularly quiet for at least 3 months prior to surgery.

Summary

It is imperative to have a thorough ocular examination with inflammatory control for at least a 3-month period, whether it be with the assistance of immunomodulatory therapy or short-term corticosteroids, to avoid complications and ensure best visual outcome.

References

1. Yamane Cde L, Vianna RN, Cardoso GP, Deschênes J, Burnier MN Jr. Cataract extraction using the phacoemulsification technique in patients with uveitis [in Portugese]. *Arq Bras Oftalmol.* 2007;70:683-688.

2. Rojas B, Foster CS. Cataract surgery in patients with uveitis. *Curr Opin Ophthalmol.* 1996;7:11-16.
3. Matsuo T, Takahashi M, Inoue Y, Egi K, Kuwata Y, Yamaoka A. Ocular attacks after phacoemulsification and intraocular lens implantation in patients with Behçet's disease. *Ophthalmologica.* 2001;215:179-182.
4. Harper SL, Foster CS. Intraocular lens explantation in uveitis. *Int Ophthalmol Clin.* 2000;40:107-116.

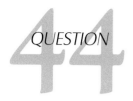

How Do I Decide When to Place an Intraocular Lens Implant in a Patient With Uveitis?

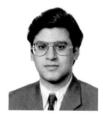

Khayyam Durrani, MD

Cataract surgery in uveitic patients is more complicated than surgery performed in patients without a history of uveitis. Even low-grade inflammation can result in chronic macular edema, optic neuropathy, and secondary glaucoma and can preclude a good visual outcome. Intraocular lens (IOL) implantation in uveitics may result in persistent inflammation, deposition of giant cells on the lens surface, perilenticular membrane formation with ciliary body dysfunction and detachment, hypotony, chronic macular edema, and, if left untreated, phthisis. IOL explantation was required in many patients due to these complications.[1] Historically, primary and even secondary IOL implantation was therefore not performed in most uveitics undergoing cataract extraction.

Advances in surgical technique, instrumentation, and lens design, as well as an increasing intolerance by ophthalmologists to low-grade inflammation in patients with uveitis during the past 25 years, have markedly improved surgical outcomes. We now perform primary IOL implantation in almost all adult patients with uveitis, provided all efforts have been made to establish the underlying diagnosis of uveitis and to treat this optimally, and inflammation is meticulously controlled for at least 3 months prior to surgery.[2] In selected cases such as in patients with chronic, granulomatous, anterior forms of uveitis as occurs in patients with sarcoidosis or Behçet's disease, some experts prefer delayed implantation of a secondary IOL. This is in contrast to patients with a history of acute, posterior, nongranular uveitis, such as in serpiginous choroiditis, presumed ocular histoplasmosis syndrome, or acute posterior multifocal placoid pigment epitheliopathy (APMPPE), in which most practitioners seem to agree that primary IOL implantation carries a lower risk of complications. Comparative outcomes of primary versus secondary IOL implantation in these disease entities, however, have not been well studied to date.

In patients with noninfectious uveitis, control of inflammation prior to surgery entails the use of perioperative corticosteroids with or without supplemental immunosuppression. The choice of prophylactic therapy would depend on the patient's diagnosis, severity of inflammation in the past, and the proximity of the patient's last flare-up of uveitis to the anticipated surgical date. Patients with a history of a single episode of mild idiopathic anterior uveitis 1 year prior to surgery, for example, may only require prednisolone acetate 1% every 4 hours for 1 week prior to and following surgery, with a subsequent taper to discontinuation over the ensuing 6 weeks. In contrast, a patient with Behçet's disease resulting in panuveitis 6 months prior to surgery would require immunomodulatory therapy resulting in quiescence for at least 3 months, with an additional 0.5 mg/kg of oral systemic corticosteroid daily, during the week prior to surgery, in addition to the topical regimen described previously. Depending on the severity of prior inflammation and recalcitrance to treatment, one may also administer 1 mg/kg of intravenous methylprednisolone on the day of surgery. In selected patients, an increased dose of the immunomodulatory "cocktail" that successfully induced remission would also be considered, allowing for adequate time for this to take effect. An alternative to systemic prophylaxis that has not been well studied is administration of periocular depot triamcinolone acetonide 3 to 4 days prior to surgery in patients known not to be steroid responders. Perioperative antimicrobial prophylaxis is administered in patients with a history of infectious uveitis with latent disease. This includes, for example, the prevention of reactivation of herpes simplex virus (HSV) uveitis with acyclovir or that of toxoplasma retinochoroiditis with pyrimethamine and sulfadiazine. With preventive measures such as these, most adult uveitic patients now undergo cataract surgery with primary IOL implantation, and reports to date indicate an excellent long-term visual prognosis.

The type of IOL that should be employed in uveitics has also been a subject of controversy. Outcomes following IOL implantation have been extensively studied, and current data indicate that in-the-bag implantation of acrylic and heparin surface-modified lenses perform better in uveitic eyes than other lens types.[3]

In contrast to adults, the timing and feasibility of IOL implantation in pediatric patients with uveitis, however, is still under debate. Primary IOL implantation was deferred in most patients with JIA-associated uveitis, and contact lens correction or aphakic spectacles were prescribed. Although most patients tolerated this surprisingly well, a substantial number, particularly in younger age groups, were unable to comply with these measures, placing them at increased risk of amblyopia and strabismus.

More recent studies suggest similar levels of postoperative inflammation and visual acuities in selected patients with JIA undergoing cataract extraction with or without IOL implantation.[4] Reports also suggest similar outcomes in children with JIA and nonJIA-associated uveitis undergoing primary IOL implantation. Careful selection of patients with pediatric uveitis must be performed. In addition to the considerations described above for adults with uveitis, factors that must be weighed in the pediatric population are patient age (older patients tend to have better outcomes), diagnosis (patients with JIA-associated uveitis are still considered to be at higher risk for IOL intolerance), degree of inflammation (a history of severe uveitis in the past may be predictive of violent postoperative inflammation), preoperative visual acuity (patients with lower acuity may experience less substantial improvements in vision), therapy at the time of surgery (patients undergoing immunosuppression likely had severe or recalcitrant uveitis in the past, and therefore have poorer outcomes), and the presence of posterior segment pathology (this may limit improvement in postoperative visual acuity). In carefully selected patients, IOL implantation may be performed in pediatric patients with uveitis with excellent outcomes.

References

1. Harper SL, Foster CS. Intraocular lens explantation in uveitis. *Int Ophthalmol Clin.* 2000;40:107-116.
2. Van Gelder RN, Leveque TK. Cataract surgery in the setting of uveitis. *Curr Opin Ophthalmol.* 2009;20:42-45.
3. Trocme SD, Li H. Effect of heparin-surface-modified intraocular lenses on postoperative inflammation after phacoemulsification: a randomized trial in a United States patient population. Heparin-Surface-Modified Lens Study Group. *Ophthalmology.* 2000;107:1031-1037.
4. Quinones K, Cervantes-Castaneda RA, Hynes AY, Daoud YJ, Foster CS. Outcomes of cataract surgery in children with chronic uveitis. *J Cataract Refract Surg.* 2009;35:725-731.

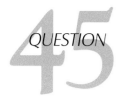

How Do I Evaluate and Treat a Patient With Persistent Inflammation Following Intraocular Surgery?

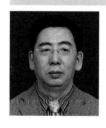

Zhi Jian Li, MD
(co-authored with John J. Huang, MD)

Persistent inflammation following intraocular surgery has a clinical presentation distinctly different from that of acute postoperative endophthalmitis. The inflammation typically consists of persistent or recurrent episodes of low-grade anterior chamber and vitreous inflammation, mild decrease in visual acuity, and conjunctival injection, and it may be associated with cystoid macula edema. Persistent inflammation following intraocular surgery can be organized into noninfectious and infectious etiologies. Prior to any aggressive intervention for noninfectious etiologies, we will rule out infectious causes through a careful examination, diagnostic work-up, and laboratory testing.

Persistent noninfectious inflammation can be autoimmune, associated with a variety of systemic and ocular-specific inflammatory conditions. Additional etiologies include uveitis-glaucoma-hyphema (UGH) syndrome, which is associated with the irritation induced by a poorly positioned anterior or posterior chamber lens against the iris or the ciliary process (Figure 45-1). Often, retained cortical or nuclear fragments in the angle, behind the iris, and in the vitreous can also cause chronic inflammation as well (see Figure 45-1).

Careful ophthalmic examination is the key to determining these potential causes. A haptic impinging on the iris or ciliary body and retained cortical material in the angle will be difficult to visualize on slit-lamp exam. Gonioscopy and ultrasound biomicroscopy are needed for diagnosis. Ultrasound evaluation of the globe should be performed if significant media opacity prevents an adequate view of the fundus or the retained cortical material in the vitreous. Surgical repositioning or exchange of intraocular lens

Figure 45-1. Partially dislocated anterior chamber intraocular lens with persistent low-grade inflammation.

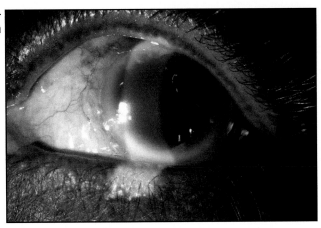

(IOL) is needed to manage patients with UGH syndrome. I often observe a small retained lens fragment while treating the inflammation and intraocular pressure medically. On the contrary, larger lens fragments require urgent pars plana vitrectomy and lensectomy.

Work-up of an autoimmune etiology should begin with a thorough review of the systems, medications, and past medical and ocular history. A focused laboratory testing is used to evaluate underlying systemic and ocular autoimmune conditions. We commonly send patients for autoimmune testing, including erythrocyte sedimentation rate (ESR), C-reactive protein (CRP) human leukocyte antigen (HLA)-B27, angiotensin-converting enzyme (ACE), antinuclear antibody (ANA), rheumatoid factor, and antineutrophil cytoplasmic antibody. Patients with an underlying systemic autoimmune disease require aggressive postoperative care, including periocular triamcinolone or oral prednisone therapy. Due to the chronic nature of the inflammation, I often give these autoimmune-mediated uveitis patients a periocular triamcinolone injection. Equally important is the preoperative, intraoperative, and postoperative management of the contralateral eye during future surgery.

Chronic infectious endophthalmitis is usually caused by less virulent organisms, such as *Propionibacterium acnes*, *Staphylococcus epidermis*, and fungal species. *P. acnes* is the most commonly isolated organism in cases of chronic infectious endophthalmitis. It begins as granulomatous corneal precipitates, hypopyon, and white or creamy plaques on the posterior capsule or IOL, weeks to months after cataract surgery, and is responsive to topical steroid treatment. The uveitis then tends to worsen as steroid is tapered. The diagnosis of *P. acnes* infection in pseudophakic endophthalmitis can be difficult due to the low yield of an anterior chamber tap with gram stain and culture. Polymerase chain reaction (PCR) is a more sensitive method than culturing to detect intraocular *P. acnes* infection in aqueous and vitreous samples.

Staphylococcus epidermidis is another pathogen that is frequently involved in chronic postoperative bacterial endophthalmitis (Figure 45-2). *S. epidermidis* can adhere to and proliferate on IOLs, and a higher degree of adhesion to silicone than to polymethylmethacrylate IOLs was found. *S. epidermidis* endophthalmitis can cause loss of integrity of the intraocular contents as a result of toxins and enzymes by both the organism and the host immune system. Culturing of intraocular fluid (aqueous and vitreous) specimens obtained by direct aspiration is critical to the proper diagnosis (see Figure 45-2).

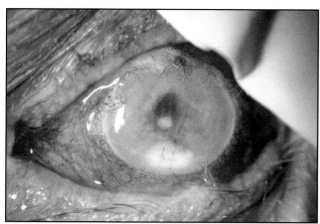

Figure 45-2. Patient with recent corneal perforation and repair demonstrating persistent anterior segment inflammation. Examination of the posterior chamber IOL revealed an infectious plaque on the anterior lens capsule.

Fungal endophthalmitis often presents in a similar clinical picture to *P. acnes* endophthalmitis, including a delayed time to the initial onset of endophthalmitis and a slow progressive course after surgery. Clinical signs include persistent corneal edema and a mass in the iris or ciliary body. Pathognomonic findings are "fluff balls" or "pearl-on-a-string" in the vitreous. Anterior chamber or vitreous tap for fungal staining and culture is needed for the proper diagnosis.

Early diagnosis and treatment with antimicrobial therapy are fundamental to optimize visual outcomes in infectious endophthalmitis. Anterior chamber paracentesis and/or diagnostic vitrectomy should be performed to obtain the maximum volume of sample for microbial staining, culture, and PCR analysis. We recommend broad-spectrum antimicrobial therapy while awaiting diagnostic results. Vancomycin (1.0 mg/0.1 mL) for gram-positive coverage, in combination with ceftazidime (2.25 mg/0.1 mL) for gram-negative coverage, is commonly used intraocularly for broad-spectrum empirical coverage. In patients with drug sensitivity to ceftazidime, amikacin (400 µg/0.1 mL) can be use in place of ceftazidime. Systemic treatment with third- and fourth-generation fluoroquinolones (eg, levofloxacin and moxifloxacin), with their broad-spectrum activity and superior intraocular penetration, may be added to the local therapy.

The treatment of fungal endophthalmitis is highly dependent on severity of disease. Fluconazole and amphotericin B are traditional first-line antifungal agents. Ocular penetration of fluconazole is good. Systemic treatment with oral fluconazole 400 mg daily may be effective for a variety of *Candida* species-associated endophthalmitis. In patients in whom the disease is unresponsive to oral therapy, intravitreal injection of amphotericin B (5 to 10 µg/0.1 mL) is highly effective for all fungal species. A new treatment option is voriconazole—both intravitreal injection of 25 µg/mL and systemic treatment provide high therapeutic levels in the eye with no evidence of retinal toxicity in both animal studies and recent case series of fungal endophthalmitis.

Pars plana vitrectomy is a crucial tool in the diagnostic process in guiding our therapy for infectious endophthalmitis. The procedure allows for a relatively large sample volume to be obtained for staining, culture, and PCR analysis. In patients with *P. acnes* endophthalmitis, partial capsulectomy is recommended in order to completely eradicate the organism from the loculated lens capsule. This treatment strategy allows removal of localized plaque material while leaving enough capsular support for the IOL. If the infection persists, a total capsulectomy with suture-fixated IOL or complete IOL exchange is recommended.

Suggested Readings

Cooper BA, Holekamp NM, Bohigian G, Thompson PA. Case-control study of endophthalmitis after cataract surgery comparing scleral tunnel and clear corneal wounds. *Am J Ophthalmol.* 2003;136:300-305.

Kunimoto DY, Kaiser RS. Incidence of endophthalmitis after 20- and 25-gauge vitrectomy. *Ophthalmology.* 2007;114:2133-2137.

Lalwani GA, Flynn HW Jr, Scott IU, et al. Acute-onset endophthalmitis after clear corneal cataract surgery (1996-2005). Clinical features, causative organisms, and visual acuity outcomes. *Ophthalmology.* 2008;115:473-476.

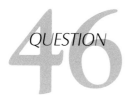

WHAT IS THE TYPICAL CLINICAL PRESENTATION OF A PATIENT WITH INTRAOCULAR LYMPHOMA?

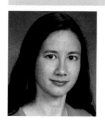

Wendy M. Smith, MD
(co-authored with H. Nida Sen, MD, MHSc)

Intraocular lymphoma is a rare entity, although the incidence in the United States has increased 3-fold during the past 2 decades.[1] Lymphoma can manifest in the eye as a primary malignancy of the retina, the vitreous, and the choroid, in which case it is called primary intraocular lymphoma (PIOL). It can also occur secondarily as a metastasis from an invasive systemic disease. Here, we are going to focus on PIOL, a subset of primary central nervous system lymphoma (PCNSL), which is typically a B-cell non-Hodgkin's lymphoma. Approximately 2000 to 3000 patients are diagnosed with PCNSL each year in the United States.[2] At the time of initial diagnosis, there may not be any other focus of lymphoma outside the eye; however, 50% to 80% of PIOL patients will go on to develop central nervous system (CNS) involvement. The median survival of PCNSL patients is 1 to 4 years depending on treatment, so it is important to make the diagnosis as soon as possible in order to initiate appropriate therapy.[3]

The diagnosis of intraocular lymphoma is often delayed due to its similarity to chronic posterior uveitis. When you approach a patient with vision loss and ocular inflammation, you should keep a high index of suspicion for intraocular lymphoma, especially if the uveitis is resistant to steroid treatment and the patient is older than 50 years of age. The typical patient will be male or female between the ages of 50 and 70 years with no previous history of uveitis. If the patient is younger, he or she might have a history of immunosuppression or immunodeficiency. There is no racial predominance. The vision loss is often gradual, progressive, painless, and accompanied by an increase in floaters. The eyes are usually quiet without pain or photophobia. Initially, only one eye may be symptomatic, but eventually up to 75% to 80% of cases are bilateral. A less common

Figure 46-1. Hazy vitritis (OD) in a 67-year-old Asian man with a history of treated biopsy-proven PCNSL prior to development of ocular symptoms. Intraocular lymphoma was confirmed with a vitreous tap.

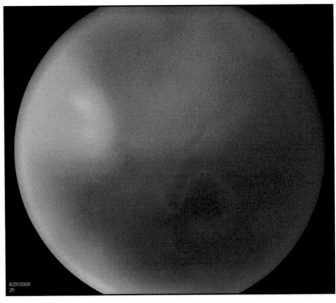

symptom is metamorphopsia. If there is preceding or concurrent CNS involvement, the patient may experience neurological symptoms, such as changes in personality or mental status, new-onset seizures, hemiparesis, or ataxia. Patients may have no visual complaints if the diagnosis of CNS lymphoma has precipitated the ophthalmic exam.

On exam, the most characteristic finding is a hazy vitritis with sheets and clumps of vitreous cells (Figure 46-1). Anterior chamber reaction is usually absent or mild with nongranulomatous keratic precipitates and aqueous cell and flare. In the posterior segment, you might observe scattered white retinal lesions or multiple cream-colored sub-retinal or sub-retinal pigment epithelium (RPE) infiltrates that may mimic sarcoidosis, viral retinitis, or a white dot syndrome. As the sub-RPE infiltrates enlarge and coalesce, multiple overlying pigment epithelium detachments may convey a "leopard spot" appearance (Figure 46-2).[3] If the sub-RPE lesions spontaneously regress, the remaining atrophic scars can resemble the "punched-out" lesions seen in presumed ocular histoplasmosis, sarcoidosis, or the geographic atrophy found in many degenerative or postinflammatory conditions (Figure 46-3). Fluorescein angiography (FA) may reveal hypofluorescent areas due to blocking by the sub-RPE lesions and hyperfluorescence from subretinal lesions or window defects in areas of atrophy (Figure 46-4; also see Figure 46-2). Interestingly, cystoid macular edema is uncommon in PIOL, and patients may have disproportionately good vision in contrast to the degree of vitritis and retinitis. Table 46-1 summarizes the common and rare findings.

The inflammation associated with PIOL may initially respond to steroid treatment because the majority of vitreous cells are "reactive" lymphocytes. Eventually, the disease will recur and progress despite steroids. To confirm the clinical suspicion of PIOL, you must obtain ocular fluid (preferably a vitreous biopsy via tap or vitrectomy) or a chorio-retinal biopsy for examination by an experienced cytopathologist. Careful handling of the specimen is crucial in order to obtain accurate results from immunohistochemical and flow cytometric studies. Testing for cytokines interleukin (IL)-10 and IL-6 as well as for immunoglobulin heavy chain (IgH) gene rearrangements can be very informative,

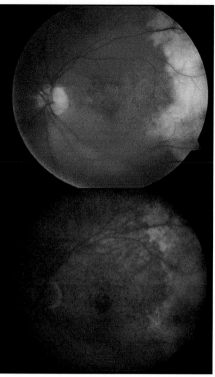

Figure 46-2. A 67-year-old man with a 15-week history of decreased vision in the left eye. Visual acuity was 20/32. Color fundus photo shows macular mottling and large cream/white subretinal lesion temporally. Fluorescein angiography shows hyperfluorescence of the subretinal lesion and small areas of hypofluorescence throughout the macula. Note the spotty "leopard-skin"-like appearance on the fluorescein angiogram.

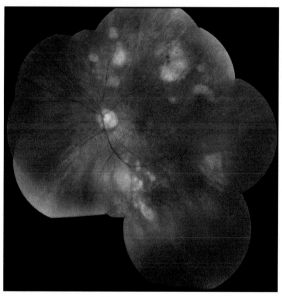

Figure 46-3. A 52-year-old woman with a 1-year history of decreased vision and choroidal lesions. Best-corrected visual acuity was 20/25 in the right and 20/800 in the left (seen in Figure 46-2). Color fundus montage shows actively appearing subretinal lesions superior to disc and atrophic "punched out" areas inferiorly.

Figure 46-4. Color fundus photos with correlating fluorescein angiography in the right and left eyes of a patient with PIOL. In the upper panel, there is hyperfluorescence from infiltrates and window defects. The lower panel shows a large hypofluorescent area due to blocking from a subretinal lesion as well as smaller hyperfluorescent infiltrates.

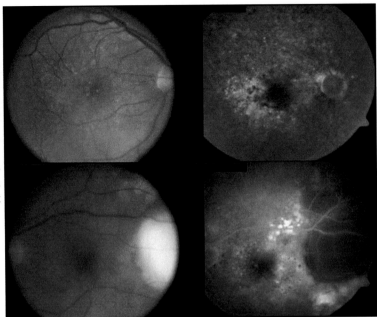

Table 46-1

Clinical Signs of Intraocular Lymphoma (From Most Common to Least)

Vitreous cells
Vitreous haze
Retinal and subretinal infiltration
Multifocal chorioretinal infiltration
Anterior chamber cells
Unifocal chorioretinal infiltration
Exudative retinal detachment
Intermediate uveitis with or without snowballs
RPE detachment
Elevated intraocular pressure
Retinal vessel occlusion
Choroidal neovascularization
Retinal neovascularization
Hypopyon

Adapted from Wakefield D, Zierhut M. Intraocular lymphoma: more questions than answers. *Ocular Immunology & Inflammation*. 2009;17:6-10.

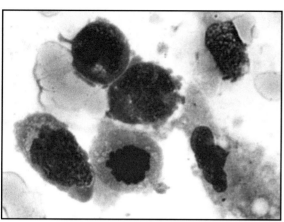

Figure 46-5. Vitreous biopsy from a patient with PIOL. The lymphoma cells are large with scant basophilic cytoplasm, large, multi-lobulated nuclei, and prominent nucleoli (Giemsa). (Reprinted with permission from Sen HN, Bodaghi B, Hoang PL, Nussenblatt R. Primary intraocular lymphoma: diagnosis and differential diagnosis. *Ocul Immunol Inflamm.* 2009;17: 133-141.)

enabling earlier diagnosis and hence earlier implementation of effective therapy. B cells secrete high levels of IL-10, whereas IL-6 is higher in uveitis. Because the majority of intraocular lymphomas are B cell-derived, a ratio of IL-10:IL-6 greater than 1.0 is highly suggestive of PIOL.[2] PCR with primers aimed at searching for IgH gene rearrangements performed on cells from the vitreous can determine if they share a common IgH gene rearrangement, thus confirming their monoclonality (another feature of lymphoma).[2] You may need multiple vitreous biopsies in order to isolate malignant cells because they can be low in number and very sensitive to steroid therapy or sample mishandling.[4] If the patient has not been previously diagnosed with PCNSL, he or she should also have a complete neurological exam, magnetic resonance imaging (MRI) of the brain and spine, and a lumbar puncture to obtain cerebrospinal fluid (CSF) for cytology. If the CSF shows malignant cells unequivocally, we don't pursue vitrectomy for diagnosis (Figure 46-5).[2]

High-dose methotrexate is the most effective treatment for PCNSL/PIOL but it is not curative. Adjunct treatments include anti-B cell therapy (rituximab, trade name Rituxan) or radiotherapy, which has the downside of severe neurologic side effects especially in patients older than 60 years of age. Even with treatment, the median survival ranges from 2 to 4 years. Patients require close monitoring with regular eye exams and MRI/light perception. Isolated ocular recurrences can be treated with an intravitreal injection of methotrexate (400 mcg/0.1 mL) and/or Rituximab (1 mg/0.1 mL). Although this does not treat or prevent CNS recurrence, in some cases, it is preferred over systemic treatment to avoid the side effects of chemotherapy or radiotherapy.

Summary

Intraocular lymphoma is classified as one of the masquerade syndromes due to its similarity to chronic posterior uveitis. In general, keep PIOL in mind in an elderly or immunocompromised patient with steroid-resistant chronic posterior uveitis, and consider further investigations for intraocular lymphoma.

References

1. Mochizuki M, Singh AD. Epidemiology and clinical features of intraocular lymphoma. *Ocul Immunol Inflamm.* 2009;17:69-72.
2. Sen HN, Bodaghi B, Hoang PL, Nussenblatt R. Primary intraocular lymphoma: diagnosis and differential diagnosis. *Ocul Immunol Inflamm.* 2009;17:133-141.
3. Choi JY, Kafkala C, Foster CS. Primary intraocular lymphoma: a review. *Semin Ophthalmol.* 2006;21:125-133.
4. Coupland SE, Chan CC, Smith J. Pathophysiology of retinal lymphoma. *Ocul Immunol Inflamm.* 2009;17:227-237.

The opinions expressed in this chapter are those solely of the authors and do not represent the views or official policies of the National Eye Institute or the United States National Institutes of Health.

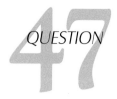
WHAT ARE THE CAUSES OF SCLEROUVEITIS?

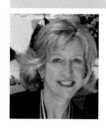

Maite Sainz de la Maza, MD

Scleritis is a severe inflammatory condition that is characterized by edema and cell infiltration of the sclera and episclera. Without treatment, the inflammatory process may extend to the adjacent tissues, causing several ocular complications, including uveitis. Long-standing uveitis may cause cataract, glaucoma, or macular edema that may lead to loss of vision. Fraunfelder and Watson[1] found that 68% of 30 enucleated eyes with a primary histological diagnosis of scleritis had signs of having had uveitis, primarily anterior. The main reason for these enucleations was pain associated with decrease in vision. Wilhelmus et al,[2] in their series of 100 enucleated eyes with a primary histological diagnosis of scleritis, found that 63% had anterior uveitis. These findings suggest that the presence of anterior uveitis in the course of scleritis could be regarded as an ominous sign because it indicates extension of scleral inflammation, which may cause complications leading to progressive decrease of vision and even loss of the eye.

In my experience, uveitis accompanying scleritis usually ranges from mild to moderate intensity, always related to the presence of active scleritis usually after some time of scleral disease, and subsides after halting scleral inflammation (Figure 47-1). Patients with sclerouveitis have more necrotizing scleritis (Figure 47-2), decrease in vision, peripheral ulcerative keratitis, and glaucoma than do patients with scleritis without uveitis.[3] Therefore, extension of scleral inflammation to the anterior uveal tract is a consequence of a more severe disease with possible ocular complications that may cause progressive visual loss.

It may occasionally be difficult to clinically distinguish primary anterior uveitis from scleritis with secondary anterior uveitis. However, vascular congestion associated with anterior uveitis typically is perilimbal, whereas vascular congestion associated with scleritis typically is either diffuse or sectorial, depending on the type of scleritis. Pathogenetic processes of primary anterior uveitis and secondary anterior uveitis after primary scleritis also are different. Primary anterior uveitis (eg, in

Figure 47-1. Patient with secondary anterior uveitis 3+ (0 to 4+) associated with scleritis in relapsing polychondritis. The patient had necrotizing scleritis and was severely inflamed, needing systemic and topical anti-inflammatory therapy. No presence of anterior uveitis before the onset of the scleritis was detected.

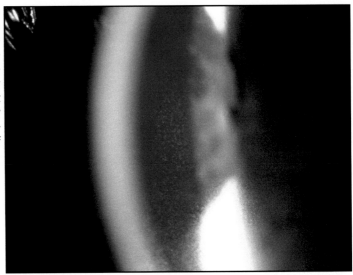

Figure 47-2. The same patient as in Figure 47-1 with very active necrotizing scleritis.

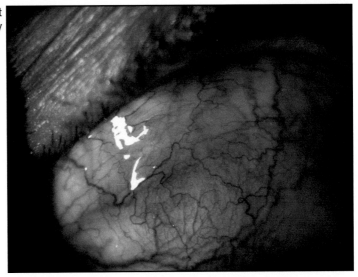

spondyloarthropathies), could be the result of the interaction between genetically controlled mechanisms (human leukocyte antigen (HLA)-B27 gene) and environmental factors (gram-negative bacterial infection), leading to immune-mediated uveal inflammation. Secondary anterior uveitis after scleritis is the result of the extension of the immune-mediated scleral inflammation.

Scleritis may be a manifestation of a potentially life-threatening systemic disease (Table 47-1). In my experience, anterior uveitis in scleritis is not more common in a patient with a particular systemic disease.[3] In the series of McGavin and associates,[4] 28% of the eyes with scleritis and rheumatoid arthritis had anterior uveitis, and 20% of the eyes with scleritis without rheumatoid arthritis had anterior uveitis, suggesting that anterior uveitis in patients with scleritis is not more common in patients with

Table 47-1

Systemic Diseases Associated With Scleritis

Rheumatoid arthritis

Systemic lupus erythematosus

Spondyloarthropathies*

Relapsing polychondritis

Wegener's granulomatosis

Polyarteritis nodosa

Behçet's disease

Giant cell arteritis

Cogan syndrome

*Spondyloarthropathies include ankylosing spondylitis, reactive arthritis, psoriatic arthritis, and arthritis and inflammatory bowel disease.

rheumatoid arthritis. In our series, 19% of the patients with sclerouveitis had rheumatoid arthritis, and 18% of the patients with scleritis without uveitis also had rheumatoid arthritis, suggesting that rheumatoid arthritis is not more common in patients with sclerouveitis.[3]

Also in our series, as many as 19% of the patients with sclerouveitis had rheumatoid arthritis, a disease rarely associated with anterior uveitis, and only 11% of the patients with sclerouveitis had one of the spondyloarthropathies (eg, ankylosing spondylitis, reactive arthritis, psoriatic arthritis, and arthritis and inflammatory bowel disease), diseases frequently associated with anterior uveitis; this suggests again that secondary anterior uveitis after extension of the primary scleral inflammation is a different entity from primary anterior uveitis.[3] Conversely, the presence of previous uveitis (primary anterior uveitis) in patients with sclerouveitis (secondary anterior uveitis) is associated only with the presence of a spondyloarthropathy and not with the presence of any other particular systemic disease; this emphasizes the importance of obtaining the history of previous uveitis before the onset of scleritis (Figure 47-3).[3]

Because the detection of anterior uveitis in a patient with scleritis connotes a poor ocular prognosis, I believe that the anterior uveal tract should be evaluated at every follow-up visit of a patient with scleritis, so that emergence of anterior uveitis may be detected promptly and systemic therapy instituted appropriately. Patients with sclerouveitis and previous uveitis should be studied for ankylosing spondylitis, reactive arthritis, psoriatic arthritis, arthritis, and inflammatory bowel disease.

Figure 47-3. Patient with secondary anterior uveitis 2+ (0 to 4+) associated with ankylosing spondylitis. The patient had diffuse scleritis and was moderately inflamed, needing systemic and topical anti-inflammatory therapy. There were several episodes of primary anterior uveitis before the onset of the scleritis.

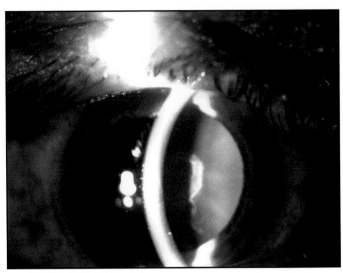

References

1. Fraunfelder FT, Watson PG. Evaluation of eyes enucleated for scleritis. *Br J Ophthalmol.* 1976;60:227-230.
2. Wilhelmus KR, Watson PG, Vasavada AR. Uveitis associated with scleritis. *Trans Ophthalmol Soc UK.* 1981;101:351-356.
3. Sainz de la Maza M, Foster CS, Jabbur NS. Scleritis-associated uveitis. *Ophthalmology.* 1997;104:58-63.
4. McGavin DDM, Williamson J, Forrester JV, et al. Episcleritis and scleritis: a study of their clinical manifestations and association with rheumatoid arthritis. *Br J Ophthalmol.* 1976;60:192-226.

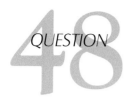

How Do I Differentiate Uveitis From Endophthalmitis?

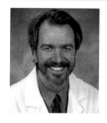

Albert T. Vitale, MD
(co-authored with Paul Yang, MD, PhD)

It is critically important to differentiate postsurgical and endogenous endophthalmitis from noninfectious uveitis, as failure to treat intraocular infection with both appropriate antimicrobial and anti-inflammatory agents may have devastating visual and systemic consequences (Figure 48-1). Clinical stigmata implicating an infectious agent may be subtle or absent, and the ocular exam alone may be misleading without carefully considering the clinical context of the presenting findings together with a careful history, review of systems, and a directed work-up.[1]

Postsurgical Inflammation

The timing and severity of intraocular inflammation with respect to a history of previous intraocular surgery, intravitreal injection, or open globe injury may be helpful in developing the differential diagnosis. While a low-grade anterior chamber cellular reaction is common following many intraocular procedures, moderate to severe inflammation involving both the anterior segment and vitreous accompanied by pain and decreased vision is presumed to be infectious until proven otherwise. Acute postoperative endophthalmitis usually presents within 2 to 11 days, but may also be seen weeks to months following glaucoma-filtering surgery or in eyes harboring wound abnormalities.[2] These scenarios constitute clear-cut surgical emergencies, which I manage according to the Endophthalmitis Vitrectomy Study (EVS) guidelines in the case of cataract surgery and more aggressively with a lower threshold for the use of diagnostic and therapeutic pars plana vitrectomy (PPV) and oral fourth-generation fluoroquinolones (ie, moxifloxacin) in patients with underlying diabetes or bleb-related and

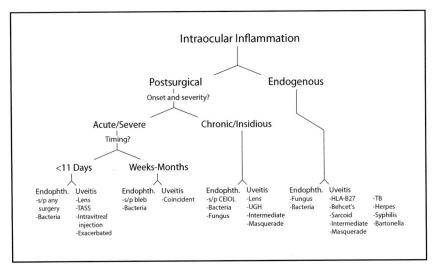

Figure 48-1. Endophthalmitis versus uveitis algorithm. (S/P indicates status post; TASS, toxic anterior segment syndrome; UGH, uveitis-glaucoma-hyphaema; HLA, human leukocyte antigen; Endophth, Endophthalmitis; TB, tuberculosis; CEIOL, cataract extraction with intraocular lens.)

post-traumatic endophthalmitis. The more challenging management decisions entail distinguishing infectious endophthalmitis from toxic, pseudo-inflammatory, and occult uveitic conditions.

Toxic anterior segment syndrome (TASS) is a sterile inflammatory reaction to contaminants in surgical devices, implants, or solutions that may arise following any anterior segment surgery and may mimic the appearance of an acute infectious endophthalmitis. While significant anterior chamber cell and flare, fibrin, and hypopyon formation may be observed in both entities, the hallmark of TASS is the brief interval between anterior segment surgery and the clinical presentation, usually within 12 to 48 hours. Signs and symptoms helpful in differentiating TASS from endophthalmitis include the characteristic appearance of diffuse (limbus-to-limbus) corneal edema (Figure 48-2), the absence of pain, and vitritis in patients with TASS. However, no clinical sign is absolute, and an infectious etiology must be ruled out if clinical suspicion remains high.

Acute infectious endophthalmitis has been reported following intravitreal injection of anti-vascular endothelial growth factor (VEGF) agents (0.03% to 0.16%) or triamcinolone acetonide (0.08% to 0.1%) and may be difficult to differentiate clinically from noninfectious pseudoendophthalmitis (0.5% to 2.0%), which is more commonly observed with both nonpreserved and preservative-free formulations or triamcinolone.[3,4] As with TASS, patients with acute noninfectious intraocular inflammation tend to present earlier (12 to 48 hours) than those with endophthalmitis, and have better vision, minimal or absent fibrin, and no pain. Free-floating triamcinolone crystals of variable sizes may be seen in the anterior chamber and settle out to form a chalk-white pseudohypopyon in contrast to the more uniform appearance of leukocytes and the yellow-white hypopyon seen in infectious cases (Figure 48-3).[4] I follow eyes with intermediate signs and symptoms after triamcinolone injection and those with even mild uveitis following intravitreal anti-VEGF therapy very closely, and manage them as infections should they progress.

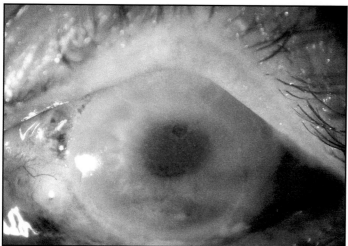

Figure 48-2. Diffuse corneal edema in TASS. (Reprinted with permission from Mamalis N, Edelhauser HF, Dawson DG, Chew J, LeBoyer RM, Werner L. Toxic anterior segment syndrome. *J Cataract Refract Surg.* 2006; 32:324-333.)

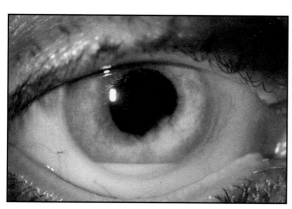

Figure 48-3. Pseudohypopyon following intravitreal injection of triamcinolone acetonide. (Reprinted with permission from DellaCroce J, Espandar L, Bernstein PS. Post-Operative Endophthalmitis. AAO 2012 Focal Points.)

A more problematic masquerade of noninfectious uveitis is chronic postoperative endophthalmitis, characterized by insidious, indolent inflammation presenting at any point in the postoperative period, but which is most often delayed weeks to months following cataract surgery, due to avirulent bacteria (*Propionibacterium acnes* [*P. acnes*], *Staphylococcus epidermidis,* and *Corynebacterium* species) or a variety of fungal pathogens. Patients with chronic postoperative endophthalmitis commonly present with fairly good vision, minimal pain, granulomatous or nongranulomatous anterior uveitis without hypopyon, keratic precipitates, and anterior vitreous cells. Bacterial infections may respond initially to topical or regional steroids only to recur once they are tapered, while progressive inflammation unresponsive to corticosteroid therapy should suggest a fungal etiology. Clinical signs that may be more indicative of a fungal etiology include the presence of a corneal infiltrate, iris or ciliary body mass, the development of necrotizing scleritis, and vitreous snowballs with a "string of pearls" appearance (Figure 48-4). While many of these findings may be seen in a variety of noninfectious entities such as intermediate uveitis, the variable response to treatment with corticosteroids alone, the presence of a white-capsular plaque representing organisms sequestered within the capsular bag (Figure 48-5), and the development of severe inflammation

Figure 48-4. "String of pearls" vitreous infiltrates in fungal endophthalmitis.

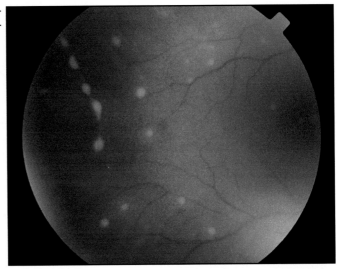

Figure 48-5. Capsular plaque in *P. acnes* endophthalmitis. (Reprinted with permission from Nick Mamalis, MD.)

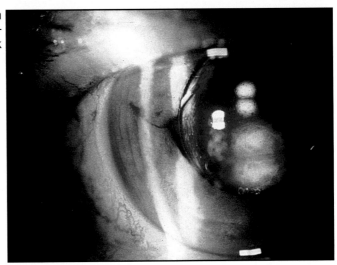

(eg, hypopyon, corneal decompensation, and frank vitritis) due to release of these organisms following YAG laser capsulotomy are clues to the diagnosis. Definitive diagnosis and treatment requires PPV, capsulectomy, and empiric intravitreal injection of antibiotics and/or antifungals with isolation of the causative organisms from gram and Giemsa stains, as well as aerobic, anaerobic, and fungal cultures obtained from undiluted vitreous and capsular plaque specimens. I instruct the lab to retain specimens for at least 2 weeks due to the slow growth of the organisms, and I routinely request polymerase chaine reaction (PCR) studies employing panbacterial and fungal primers, as well as cytology, to improve the diagnostic yield and to rule out a neoplastic masquerade. Concurrent medical treatment with oral clarithromycin or voriconazole, both of which achieve good intravitreal concentrations, may be useful adjuncts in the management of suspected chronic bacterial and fungal endophthalmitis, respectively. Failing these interventions, I perform complete capsulectomy and intraocular lens (IOL) removal to achieve a cure.

Chronic postoperative inflammation may also be due to lens-induced uveitis, which occurs in response to retained lens material in the anterior chamber or vitreous following cataract surgery, trauma to the lens capsule, or in the setting of a hypermature cataract. Lens-induced uveitis commonly presents with keratic precipitates, posterior synechiae, and elevated intraocular pressure with a variable degree of intraocular inflammation, the severity of which is related to the amount of retained lens material. Mild inflammation due to retained cortex may respond to topical or systemic corticosteroids. However, more severe inflammation, and that in the setting of trauma or hypermature cataract, require surgical removal of lens material with a low threshold for vitreous tap and injection of antibiotics should the clinical picture suggest infectious endophthalmitis.

While an uncommon complication with modern IOLs, chronic inflammation and microhyphema following cataract surgery may result from iris chafing of the edges, haptics, or footplates of the IOL and as part of the uveitis-glaucoma-hyphema (UGH) syndrome. Careful evaluation of the type of anterior chamber cells (pigment, red blood cells, and/or leukocytes), iris transillumination defects, gonioscopy, and high-resolution ultrasound biomicroscopy of the anterior segment for evidence of lens malposition usually establishes the correct diagnosis.

Finally, chronic intraocular inflammation in the elderly, irrespective of previous intraocular surgery, should always raise the possibility of intraocular involvement from primary CNS lymphoma, the diagnosis of which requires a high degree of clinical suspicion and diagnostic PPV.

Endogenous Inflammation

Patients with pre-existing uveitis may have a severe exacerbation of intraocular inflammation within a week of surgery that may mimic an infectious etiology; however, pain, hypopyon, and fibrin are atypical of noninfectious postsurgical uveitis. Alternatively, new onset of inflammation following surgery may be unrelated to the procedure itself, heralding instead the first episode of uveitis from other causes. For example, most patients with human leukocyte antigen (HLA)-B27-associated acute, nongranulomatous anterior uveitis present with characteristic signs and symptoms that make the diagnosis without invasive laboratory confirmation; however, a subgroup of these patients may present with a severe panuveitis mimicking infectious endophthalmitis.[5] Similarly, intermediate uveitis, Behçet's disease, ocular sarcoidosis, and infectious posterior and panuveitis due to toxoplasmosis, syphilis, herpes viridae, tuberculosis, and bartonellosis have distinctive historical features, clinical presentations, and confirmatory laboratory findings; however, in some cases, they may be difficult to distinguish from endogenous bacterial or fungal endophthalmitis, especially in the immunocompromised or elderly patient.

While an extraocular focus of infection is identifiable in the vast majority of cases of endogenous endophthalmitis, systemic signs of infection may be subtle or absent and lead to an erroneous diagnosis of an autoimmune uveitis, which, if treated with steroids alone, carries significant risk of morbidity and mortality. Patients with altered immune status, including immunologically immature neonates, are at most risk for developing endogenous endophthalmitis. Predisposing conditions include immunosuppressive therapy, AIDS, diabetes, systemic malignancy or autoimmune disease, sickle cell anemia, intravenous hyperalimentation or drug use, and recent gastrointestinal surgery. A history of recent pneumonia, periodontal or urinary tract infection, sinusitis, osteomyelitis, bacterial meningitis, or liver abscess may uncover a subtle nidus of infection.

Most cases of endogenous endophthalmitis are fungal, but a significant minority is bacterial and may present with signs and symptoms similar to those of autoimmune uveitis or an infectious posterior or panuveitis. Bacterial infection usually presents acutely with pain, photophobia, and severe vision loss. Ocular findings include periorbital and lid edema, elevated intraocular pressure (IOP; characteristic of other infectious uveitis due to herpes, toxoplasmosis, and syphilis), anterior chamber fibrin and hypopyon, and vitritis. Roth spots and retinal microabscesses may be seen in both bacterial and fungal endogenous endophthalmitis. In contrast, fungal infection develops more slowly with focal or multifocal areas of white or creamy chorioretinitis, which may break through into the vitreous, producing localized cellular condensations over the site. Vitreous "fluff balls" in a "string of pearls" configuration, especially when localized over the posterior pole, as opposed to the anterior or inferior vitreous base as seen in ocular sarcoidosis or intermediate uveitis, are suggestive but certainly not specific for fungal infection (see Figure 48-4).

Culture results from blood and other bodily fluids together with ocular culture and PCR analysis of specimens obtained following diagnostic PPV and/or retinal biopsy and empiric intravitreal medications as described above establish the diagnosis and guide subsequent therapy. Consultation with an infectious disease specialist is mandatory as systemic antimicrobial therapy may be required for prolonged periods of time and given the potential for significant morbidity. I carefully follow chorioretinal lesions due to *Candida*, which have not yet broken through to the vitreous for progression as they may be effectively treated with the oral triazole antifungal agents fluconazole or voriconazole. With more extensive vitritis, I find PPV to be therapeutic in debulking the pathogen load especially in cases of fungal endophthalmitis.

Appearances are deceiving in distinguishing endophthalmitis from uveitis. The critical importance of a detailed history and review of systems in distinguishing infectious from noninfectious intraocular inflammation, in guiding the appropriate workup and subsequent therapy, especially in the diagnosis of endogenous endophthalmitis, cannot be overstated.

References

1. Foster CS, Vitale AT. *Diagnosis and Treatment of Uveitis*. Philadelphia, PA: WB Saunders Company; 2002.
2. Lemley GA, Han DP. Endophthalmitis: a review of current evaluation and management. *Retina*. 2007;27: 662-680.
3. Mezad-Koursh D, Goldstein M, Heilwail G, et al. Clinical characteristics of endophthalmitis after an injection of intravitreal antivascular endothelial growth factor. *Retina*. 2010;30:1051-1057.
4. Roth DB, Flynn HW Jr. Distinguishing between infectious and noninfectious endophthalmitis after intravitreal triamcinolone injection. *Am J Ophthalmol*. 2008;146:346-347.
5. Sanghvi C, Mercieca K, Jones NP. Very severe HLA-B27-associated panuveitis mimicking endophthalmitis: a case series. *Ocul Immunol Inflamm*. 2010;18:139-141.

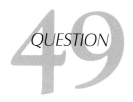

SHOULD I ENUCLEATE THE INCITING EYE
IN A PATIENT WITH SYMPATHETIC OPHTHALMIA?

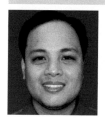

Jose Cuevas Francisco III, MD
(co-authored with Harvey Siy Uy, MD)

Sympathetic ophthalmia (SO) is a bilateral, granulomatous, panuveitis precipitated by penetrating trauma to the inciting/exciting eye resulting in an inflammatory response in the uninjured, sympathizing eye. SO is a potential, bilaterally blinding complication of open globe injury or ocular surgery.[1] Vision loss may result from cataract, secondary glaucoma, maculopathy, retinal detachment, optic neuritis, vasculitis, or neovascularization. It is believed that penetrating trauma allows ocular antigens to gain access to lymphatics and be presented to the systemic immune system, producing self-destructive, autoimmune, ocular sequelae.

With improvements in trauma and surgical care, SO has become a rare, though still feared, uveitic condition. The diagnosis of SO should be suspected in patients with recent history of penetrating trauma or surgery and bilateral panuveitis. The onset of SO may be insidious with symptoms manifesting a few weeks to several months or years after the inciting injury. The vast majority (90%) of cases manifest within a year of injury.

SO presents classically as granulomatous panuveitis. The range of intraocular signs include anterior uveitis (Figure 49-1) with mutton fat keratic precipitates, moderate to severe vitritis, white-yellow chorioretinal infiltrates called Dalen-Fuchs nodules (Figure 49-2), and papillitis. Systemic involvement may include Vogt-Koyanagi-Harada (VKH) syndrome-like findings such as alopecia, vitiligo, poliosis, dysacousia, and cerebrospinal fluid pleiocytosis. The vision-robbing complications of SO are legion and include cataracts; secondary glaucoma; cystoid macular edema; retinal detachment; optic neuritis; retinal vasculitis; subretinal fibrosis; and atrophy of the retina, choroid, and optic nerve (Figures 49-3 and 49-4).

Figure 49-1. Slit-lamp photograph demonstrating iris nodules and posterior synechiae in a patient with sympathetic ophthalmia.

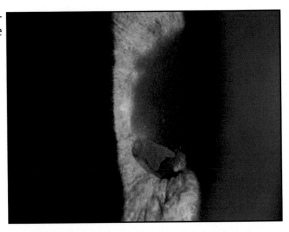

Figure 49-2. Fundus photograph demonstrating peripheral yellow-white choroidal lesions (Dalen-Fuchs nodules) in a patient with sympathetic ophthalmia.

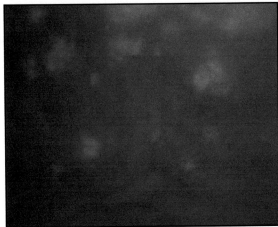

Figure 49-3. Fundus photograph demonstrating multiple chorioretinal scars and subretinal fibrosis following penetrating trauma in the inciting eye of a patient with sympathetic ophthalmia.

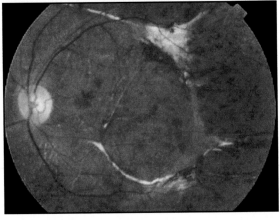

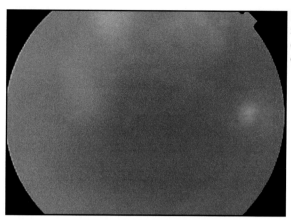

Figure 49-4. Fundus photograph demonstrating severe vitritis and inferior retinal detachment in the sympathizing, contralateral eye of the patient in Figure 49-3.

The only certain prevention for SO is enucleation, which should ideally be performed within 2 weeks of ocular injury. Mere evisceration may still lead to SO as postevisceration uveal antigens may still remain and incite an autoimmune response.

In our practice, however, I do not routinely enucleate the inciting eye as a means for preventing SO. The reasons for my approach are 1) current microsurgical techniques for ocular surgery or repair of ocular trauma have led to a decrease in the incidence of SO, 2) the advent of intraocular and systemic immunomodulatory agents have greatly improved the prognosis of SO, and 3) the inciting or exciting eyes sometimes have better visual outcomes than sympathizing eyes. In the Vietnam, Korean, and Arab-Israeli Six-Day War, no cases of SO were reported. This suggests that improved management of ocular trauma, including use of antibiotics, corticosteroids, and microsurgical repair, have decreased the risk for SO.

Enucleation remains a controversial approach. While some authors have suggested that early enucleation of the exciting eye led to improved visual prognosis, Kilmartin and associates suggested that enucleation of the inciting eye following onset of SO did not lead to a better visual outcome in the sympathizing eye nor lessened the need for immunosuppressive therapy.[1,2] No clinical trials have compared the outcomes of these 2 opposite approaches.

Despite a chronic, relapsing course, good outcomes may be obtained with immunosuppressive agents or immunomodulatory therapy (IMT). Patients with acute SO should be promptly started on systemic corticosteroids (eg, prednisone 1 to 2 mg/kg/day). Using this approach, Makley and Azar reported that 65% of eyes had 20/60 or better visual acuity.[3] Supplementation of systemic corticosteroids with periocular corticosteroid depot (eg, trans-septal triamcinolone acetonide 40 mg/1 mL) may provide additional, rapid immunosuppressive effect.

Severe or recurrent cases will require combination therapy with one or more immunosuppressive agents. Cyclophosphamide, cyclosporine, azathioprine, and methotrexate are frequently used corticosteroid-sparing drugs. I thoroughly discuss the potential risks and benefits of enucleation versus IMT side effects prior to initiation of any treatment and regularly monitor patients for treatment-related side effects. Co-management with an internist or rheumatologist should be considered when the ophthalmologist is not trained in the use of IMT. The introduction of biologic drugs and sustained-release ocular implants for the treatment of SO may further lead to reduced rates of enucleation.[4] Despite the availability of nonsurgical methods of treatment, the long-term prognosis for SO is variable, and poor vision may be the end result despite IMT.

I reserve enucleation of the inciting eye when it is blind, painful, phthsical, or disfigured. Enucleation in these cases may provide pain relief and improved cosmesis after fitting ocular prostheses. Inadequate access to health care or poor compliance with IMT medications are factors to consider when choosing a surgical versus medical approach to treatment.

Summary

Fortunately, SO is becoming an extremely rare complication of penetrating ocular trauma. Enucleation of the inciting eye can usually be avoided by early recognition of SO and prompt, sustained institution of corticosteroids and IMT. In occasional instances, enucleation may be considered for blind, painful, and disfigured inciting eyes.

References

1. Kilmartin DJ, Dick AD, Forrester JV. Prospective surveillance of sympathetic ophthalmia in the United Kingdom and Republic of Ireland. *Br J Ophthalmol.* 2000;84:259-263.
2. Lubin JR, Albert DM, Weinstein M. Sixty-five years of sympathetic ophthalmia. A clinicopathologic review of 105 cases (1913-1978). *Ophthalmology.* 1980;87:109-121.
3. Makley TA, Azar A. Sympathetic ophthalmia: a long term follow up. *Arch Ophthalmol.* 1978;96:257-262.
4. Mahajan VB, Gehrs KM, Goldstein DA, Fischer DH, Lopez JS, Folk JC. Management of sympathetic ophthalmia with the fluocinolone acetonide implant. *Ophthalmology.* 2009;116:552-557.

FINANCIAL DISCLOSURES

Dr. Esen K. Akpek has no financial or proprietary interest in the materials presented herein.

Dr. Amro Ali has no financial or proprietary interest in the materials presented herein.

Dr. Sofia Androudi has no financial or proprietary interest in the materials presented herein.

Dr. Stephen D. Anesi has no financial or proprietary interest in the materials presented herein.

Dr. William Ayliffe has not disclosed any relevant financial relationships.

Dr. Neal P. Barney received a research grant from Alcon Laboratories.

Dr. Periklis Brazitikos has no financial or proprietary interest in the materials presented herein.

Dr. Nicholas J. Butler has no financial or proprietary interest in the materials presented herein.

Dr. Margarita Calonge has no financial or proprietary interest in the materials presented herein.

Dr. Chi-Chao Chan has no financial or proprietary interest in the materials presented herein.

Dr. David S. Chu is a consultant for Alcon, Allergan, Analysis Group, and Inspire. Dr. Chu has received research support from Luxbio, Novartis, and EyeGate.

Dr. Emmett T. Cunningham Jr has no financial or proprietary interest in the materials presented herein.

Dr. Mark S. Dacey is on the speaker's bureau with Allergical Pharmaceuticals for the Ozurdex intravitreal implant.

Dr. Janet L. Davis has received grant support from Santen.

Dr. Khayyam Durrani has no financial or proprietary interest in the materials presented herein.

Dr. C. Stephen Foster has not disclosed any relevant financial relationships.

Dr. Jose Cuevas Francisco III has no financial or proprietary interest in the materials presented herein.

Dr. Debra A. Goldstein has no financial or proprietary interest in the materials presented herein.

Dr. Arusha Gupta has no financial or proprietary interest in the materials presented herein.

Dr. David M. Hinkle has no financial or proprietary interest in the materials presented herein.

Dr. Gary N. Holland has no financial or proprietary interest in the materials presented herein.

Dr. John J. Huang has no financial or proprietary interest in the materials presented herein.

Dr. Henry J. Kaplan has no financial or proprietary interest in the materials presented herein.

Dr. Muhammad Kashif Israr has no financial or proprietary interest in the materials presented herein.

Dr. John H. Kempen has received research support from the National Eye Institute, Research to Prevent Blindness, and the Mackall Foundation. Dr. Kempen is an ad hoc consultant to Alcon, Allergan, Lux Biosciences, and Sanofi Pasteur.

Dr. Olivia L. Lee has no financial or proprietary interest in the materials presented herein.

Dr. Phuc Lehoang has no financial or proprietary interest in the materials presented herein.

Dr. Erik Letko has no financial or proprietary interest in the materials presented herein

Dr. Zhi Jian Li has no financial or proprietary interest in the materials presented herein.

Dr. Sue Lightman has no financial or proprietary interest in the materials presented herein.

Dr. Dorine Makhoul has no financial or proprietary interest in the materials presented herein.

Dr. Annal Dhananjayan Meleth has no financial or proprietary interest in the materials presented herein.

Dr. Elisabetta Miserocchi has no financial or proprietary interest in the materials presented herein.

Dr. Lama Mulki has no financial or proprietary interest in the materials presented herein.

Dr. Ron Neumann is an employee of Teva Pharmaceutical Industries Ltd.

Dr. Quan Dong Nguyen is a member of the scientific advisory board for Santen, Bausch and Lomb, and Lux Biosciences.

Dr. C. Mitchel Opremcak has no financial or proprietary interest in the materials presented herein.

Dr. Suzanne Katrina V. Palafox has no financial or proprietary interest in the materials presented herein.

Dr. John Randolph has no financial or proprietary interest in the materials presented herein.

Dr. Narsing A. Rao receives funding from the National Institutes of Health for uveitis reseach.

Dr. Russell W. Read has no financial or proprietary interest in the materials presented herein.

Dr. Alejandro Rodríguez-García has no financial or proprietary interest in the materials presented herein.

Dr. Manolette R. Roque has no financial or proprietary interest in the materials presented herein.

Dr. James T. Rosenbaum has no financial or proprietary interest in the materials presented herein.

Dr. Aniki Rothova has no financial or proprietary interest in the materials presented herein.

Dr. Maite Sainz de la Maza has no financial or proprietary interest in the materials presented herein.

Dr. C. Michael Samson has not disclosed any relevant financial relationships.

Dr. H. Nida Sen has no financial or proprietary interest in the materials presented herein.

Dr. Yasir J. Sepah has no financial or proprietary interest in the materials presented herein.

Dr. Rajiv Shah has no financial or proprietary interest in the materials presented herein.

Dr. Sana S. Siddique has no financial or proprietary interest in the materials presented herein.

Dr. Wendy M. Smith has no financial or proprietary interest in the materials presented herein.

Dr. Eric B. Suhler has received research support from Abbott, BMS, EyeGate, Genentech, LuxBio, Novartis, and the Department of Veterans Affairs.

Sarah Syeda has no financial or proprietary interest in the materials presented herein.

Dr. Joseph Tauber has no financial or proprietary interest in the materials presented herein.

Dr. Simon Taylor has no financial or proprietary interest in the materials presented herein.

Dr. Howard H. Tessler has no financial or proprietary interest in the materials presented herein.

Dr. Jennifer E. Thorne has no financial or proprietary interest in the materials presented herein.

Dr. Evangelia Tsironi has no financial or proprietary interest in the materials presented herein.

Dr. Harvey Siy Uy has no financial or proprietary interest in the materials presented herein.

Dr. Albert T. Vitale is a consultant for Bausch and Lomb and ACIONT.

Dr. Paul Yang has no financial or proprietary interest in the materials presented herein.

Dr. Ellen N. Yu has not disclosed any relevant financial relationships.

Dr. Manfred Zierhut has no financial or proprietary interest in the materials presented herein.

INDEX

Printed in the United States
by Baker & Taylor Publisher Services